"Never again will I hear 'ne
facing life's major challenge
Thompson. Together, they prove wnat tnese words truly mean to
those who insist on living them. Certainly true love and joy, even in
loss, are the rewards."

--Paul Linnman
Television and radio personality, Portland, OR

"Suffering is an inescapable part of life. In an age obsessed with
dignity in death, Marilyn offers a clear example of what it means to
honor God and embrace life in the midst of suffering. A serious
treatment of an emotional issue, Leave a Legacy is thought-
provoking and insightful. If you are looking for hope and comfort in
an otherwise hopeless situation, Live a Legacy will help you find God
in the midst of suffering."

--Georgene Rice, host
The Georgene Rice Show, KPDQ Radio, Portland, OR

"Although the Thompsons for months became almost a daily subject
of debate on both local and national television news, it is the story of
their life together that is so very moving…It really is quite an
amazing love story. You're laughing one minute and crying the
next. I really believe that many people who are going through
struggles, whether physical or otherwise, will find strength in her
story."

--The late Dr. Ron Mehl
Pastor and award winning author

"I'm so grateful for Marilyn's inspiring account of walking with her
husband Troy through earth's final journey. Troy faced a long fight
against Lou Gehrig's disease. Through it Marilyn exhibited
remarkable courage and hope. Troy did too. This is an amazing true
story you'll want to share with family and friends."

--David Sanford
Author of If God Disappears (Tyndale House Publishers)

Live a Legacy, Leave a Legacy

Choosing to live with hope and courage in the face of Lou Gehrig's disease

MARILYN THOMPSON

Edited by Elizabeth Jones
Cover Design by Michelle Winchester
Cover Photo by Elrike Shaw

Published by Holly Press

DEDICATION

To Troy—my loving and devoted husband, best friend, and protector. I know you're creating beautiful gardens in heaven. You certainly did here on earth, as well as in the lives of those who knew you.

"Above all else, guard your heart for it is the well spring of life."
Proverbs 4:23 (Troy's favorite scripture)

CONTENTS

Prologue
Spirit to Spirit

So few words, so much said…

The spacious foyer of our home was rapidly filling up, buzzing with activity. Reporters and cameramen arrived in groups of two and three, carrying equipment, brief cases, and clipboards. The vans lining the circular driveway each displayed a different television station's logo.

Stepping over extension cords snaked across the dark hardwood floors, I made my way around black duffel bags to the front door. Through the etched glass of the double doors, I could see more reporters waiting to be ushered in. Trying not to let my nervousness show, I shook hands and introduced myself. They all seemed to know each other, exchanging greetings with familiarity, yet with a professional politeness lacking in friendliness. Off to the side, a conversation was heating up in the dining room.

An attractive blonde woman, dressed professionally in a blue business suit, took me aside and filled me in on what was happening. She kindly explained that under the circumstances, they had all agreed to only have one camera in the bedroom, the stage for this breaking news story. All the stations would then share the film.

The heated conversation was over which station's cameraman would be chosen. Surveying the scene gave me a glimpse into the highly competitive world of news reporters.

Self-consciously, I made my way past several reporters standing in the doorway to our bedroom. Once a sanctuary of privacy and intimacy, our bedroom was now the center for a top news story that would soon make its way around the world.

My husband lay motionless in our bed, paralyzed by a devastating disease that had ravaged his body and left him unable to move or speak. His eyes, the only movement he had left, were darting back and forth, taking in what was happening around him.

As he saw me come through the door, our eyes met. A smile formed as relief washed over his face at the sight of me. For Troy, I was not only the wife who loved him beyond words, but I was also the only one in the room who could understand his slow and painstaking attempts to communicate.

Through those deep blue eyes, so much was said without words…

1
STORM CLOUDS GATHERING

"All sunshine makes a desert..."
~Troy Thompson

The morning was dragging on unusually slowly. I glanced at the clock on my computer for probably the twentieth time. Accustomed to being busy at work, I would usually wish the day would slow down so I could get more of my "to do list" done.

Today was different. I was anxiously waiting for it to be noon. It was one of the rare occasions that I was having lunch with my husband. We worked in two different towns that were an hour apart, but today Troy was on his way to Portland for a doctor's appointment, and we had made a date to meet afterward at the Olive Garden, a popular Italian restaurant. It was one of those gorgeous spring days that don't happen very often in Oregon. When they do, everyone seems to smile more, and look for excuses to head outdoors.

Troy worked on the outskirts of Salem as a landscaper for Marion County. When the new jail was built, he had the opportunity to design and install the landscaping for the jail campus.

As Ted Nelson, the jail commander, said, "He took a twenty-acre parcel of farmland and with ingenuity and hard work transformed it into a complex that would rival most golf courses and country clubs around the state."

Troy loved his job, designing and installing landscaping, working with the plants. I kept trying to convince him to start his own company and work closer to home in Lake Oswego, an hour north of Salem. But for Troy, it wasn't just about the landscaping—he knew he was in a unique position to help others, to maybe make a difference in someone's life.

Because of his strong work ethic and desire to help others, Troy had the opportunity to pioneer a program using inmates from the jail for an outside grounds crew. It wasn't difficult getting the guys to jump at a chance to be outdoors. The challenge was that a lot of them just did the bare minimum they could get away with until their next cigarette break. However, for a few, it made a real difference as they were learning a trade they could use when they got out of jail.

Troy often came to work on his days off, pulling his inmate crew out of their cellblocks. He took them down to the classroom where he would spend hour after hour, trying to teach them about landscape design and maintenance. More importantly, he taught them, through example, some important lessons about life. Unlike most inmate supervisors, Troy didn't demand work from his inmates, expecting them to do the work he didn't want to do. Instead, he asked them to work with him, and he taught them the right way to do things by doing the work with them. Day in and day out, he worked shoulder to shoulder with the inmates until the job was finished.

Troy would show up for work at 6:30 a.m., in khaki shorts and a t-shirt, and pick up his inmate crew. At the end of the day, through friendly competition, they would decide who came back with the dirtiest t-shirt. More often than not, Troy would win.

Troy treated people respectfully and with unconditional love, whether they deserved it or not. He taught the men about respect by the example of how he treated others.

Floyd was a 60-year-old man with an attitude. A big man, baldheaded and with tattoos over just about every inch of his body, Floyd was used to being in charge. He didn't like the idea of taking orders from some 30-year-old "know it all plant lover." But Troy's 6'4" frame commanded some respect of its own.

Floyd knew that it was a chance to get on the outside, to get some exercise for his once hard muscles, now showing signs of softness. His knees were starting to stiffen with arthritis.

Since Floyd's vocabulary was mostly limited to words with four letters, he and Troy didn't get off to a good start on the first day. One of Troy's rules was no cussing.

The next morning, Troy was surprised to see Floyd's name show up on his crew list again. He figured Floyd wouldn't be back. Muttering under his breath, Floyd went to work, digging the trenches for some new irrigation lines. Troy smiled to himself.

Floyd showed up the next day—and the next. In fact, he never missed a day, which was unusual in this environment. There was a lot of turnover on the crew, with some quitting and others being cut for bad behavior, or released or moved to another jail. But not Floyd.

As the weeks went by, Troy noticed a subtle change. Little things, like an occasional "thanks," from this gruff man, and occasionally, even a smile. Over time, Floyd began to surprise everyone by going the extra mile to do something he wasn't asked to.

After a while, when a new inmate came on board, it was Floyd who would be the first to say, "Hey man, don't you be talking like that. Our boss man don't like it!"

§

Then there was Morgan, another inmate at the jail. Morgan was deaf, but that wasn't the only challenge he presented. He was totally out of control upon arrival at the jail, and was almost immediately put in solitary confinement.

It didn't take Morgan long to figure out how to open a $2,000 high security door with the handle of a toothbrush. He was moved to a different cell in a different part of the jail (with a different locking mechanism!), where it didn't take him long to figure out how to dismantle and set off an $800 security sprinkler system—not once, but three times!

It didn't matter to Troy that Morgan was a security risk or that it was difficult to communicate with him because he was deaf. Troy asked if he could try an experiment and have Morgan on his outside work crew. Ted, the jail commander, was hesitant, but took a chance and agreed.

Troy went downtown to the library and checked out a book on sign language. Within a week, the two of them were communicating, in a crude sort of way. The irony was unimaginable—to think that just two years later it would be Troy learning how to communicate all over again, just to survive.

Morgan's reaction to Troy was truly remarkable. He respected Troy for putting in the extra effort. According to Ted, this inmate turned out to be one of the best inmate workers the jail has ever had. The behavior problems within the jail stopped. Ted shared, "We all learned a valuable lesson about human behavior through Troy's methods. Troy saw the potential in this man and accentuated the positive. Low and behold, the response was nothing short of miraculous."

Morgan had developed a habit of spending all of his time in and out of the jail. Whenever he was released, he would immediately commit a crime that would get him sent back. After working with Troy, the next time Morgan was released, he did not come back. Six years later, he still had not been back.

§

Pulling into the parking lot of the Olive Garden, I spotted Troy's white Toyota pickup. My heart started beating a little faster at the thought of seeing him. I hopped out of my black sports car and headed quickly to the front door, not wanting to waste any of our precious time together. There he stood in the foyer leaning up against a post, his arms folded casually across his chest, looking as handsome as ever. Even though it was early spring, his skin was already deeply tanned from working outside. He wrapped his strong arms around me and gave me a long kiss.

It was good to be together, just the two of us — no kids, no interruptions. We loved our girls, but life with four daughters was a whirlwind. Troy and I had just celebrated our two-year anniversary the month before. We still felt like newlyweds. The night he proposed seemed like yesterday...

§

The last rays of the sunset had just disappeared and the twilight was rapidly giving way to the deeper purple shades of evening. Troy and I were heading home on Highway 101 after a day at the coast.

Suddenly, Troy turned off the highway and down a side street. Without giving an explanation, he drove the couple of blocks to the beach. Pulling the car up to the edge of the sand, he shut off the engine and came around to open my door.

Taking my hand, he guided me down the short path to the beach, now barely visible as the shadows of the night were closing in.

Turning to face me, he took both my hands in his, and said he wanted us to spend the rest of our lives together. He explained that he had hardly dared to dream that he would find someone to love as much as he loved me. Then, as he started to ramble on about how this wasn't the way he planned to ask me, and how he was going to "rent a suit of armor and…" I interrupted.

"Yes! Yes I will marry you!" I couldn't believe he seemed nervous that I might not say yes! I had grown to love him just as deeply, and after being on my own raising two daughters for almost eleven years, I was thrilled to have found real love. So on that November night in 1991, we were engaged and started dreaming and planning our new life together.

Neither one of us could have imagined, at that moment, when time seemed to stand still, what was just around the corner for us.

We were married that spring on March 14, 1992. We chose that month partly because of its significance for me. It was the month that both my parents had died, my mom just the year before from a sudden and massive brain aneurism. My dad had died three years earlier after battling Parkinson's, a degenerative neurological disease. So March was not my favorite month, as it became a cruel reminder of the losses. Starting my new life with Troy helped to ease the loss of my parents and I looked forward to March becoming a month of new beginnings.

Between us we had three daughters — my two teenagers, Summer and Holly, and Troy's six-year-old daughter, Michelle (just to keep things balanced we got a male dog). And so our new life as a "blended family" began!

Six months later, we learned I was pregnant. Having more children wasn't in "the plan." Now I know that this shouldn't normally come as a surprise. But even from a medical viewpoint, this was unexpected!

I was shocked...

Troy was ecstatic!

And it was another girl.

Victoria was born June 2, 1993. This newest addition turned out to be one of the best things that could have happened. God, in his infinite wisdom, knew how much we would need her joy and bright spirit in the days and years that were ahead.

§

It was shortly after Victoria was born that Troy started having trouble with his back.

He returned to work from "maternity leave," and as he was lifting 200+ pounds of rubber hose, a twinge shot through his back. He normally had no trouble lifting this kind of weight, but this time he strained the muscle right inside the left shoulder blade.

We figured it was because he had taken off the month of June to be home with the new baby and me, and he probably got a little out of shape.

He first went to see his doctor, then a physical therapist.

I worked on massaging his back in the evenings, trying to work out the stubborn knots. We could not seem to get it back to normal.

One night, lying in bed, he told me to touch his left arm, just below the shoulder.

"Do you feel that?" he asked

"You mean that twitching?" I replied. It was just a little muscle twitch, the kind everyone gets from time to time.

"It never stops," he said quietly. "It's always there."

§

After seeing an orthopedist, and going through lots of physical therapy, his back improved some. But the twitching didn't stop. By now, nine months had passed since Troy had first started having trouble with his back. His doctor had been hopeful that the twitching would go away once the muscle injury healed. He recommended Troy go see a neurologist. "It's probably nothing, but it wouldn't hurt to get it checked out," he advised.

Our lunch date began after his visit to the neurologist. The waitress seated us at a table in the corner, next to a window. I was chattering away about my day when I noticed that Troy wasn't really listening. He was distracted, edgy. Then I remembered the doctor appointment.

"So, what happened today? What did the doctor say?" I asked.

His eyes avoided mine. I reached across the table for the saltshaker as the waitress refilled our water. Picking at his food with his fork, he took his time before answering. He told me they had run some tests. It would be two weeks before we would know anything.

"Know anything about what?" I asked. He was starting to get my attention.

"Dr. Gibbs says that this muscle twitching could be something as minor as lead poisoning or in the worst case, something called Lou Gehrig's disease," Troy replied, still not looking at me. My fork stopped halfway to my mouth.

"What do you mean lead poisoning? How did you get lead poisoning?! They can treat that, right?" I fired off the questions, not waiting for his answers.

It did not even occur to me to consider the worst-case scenario. I was focused in on the lead poisoning, hopeful they were wrong about that. Probably the tests would show that there was nothing wrong, I told myself.

"Have you ever heard of Lou Gehrig's disease?" Troy asked. No, I hadn't.

"Me either," he said.

I could tell from Troy's unusually quiet mood that he was a lot more concerned about this than he wanted to let on. Something the doctor said had given him reason to think this may be far more serious than lead poisoning. But he wasn't sharing that with me.

We would have to wait. Two weeks. Two long weeks...

2
A MOTHER'S LOVE

"Children and mothers never truly part —
Bound in the beating of each other's heart."
~Charlotte Gray

    The following day was Saturday. Troy had plans to spend a long-awaited weekend with Michelle at our beach house. Troy was really looking forward to spending some one-on-one time with his daughter at our peaceful retreat. Michelle, now eight, lived with her mom and step-dad in Salem. It tore him up that he didn't get to see her more. She would come and spend every other weekend with us in our chaos of teenagers, a toddler, assorted friends and of course, the dog.

    With all these wonderful distractions, an eight-year-old naturally wanted to hang out with her new sisters. She especially looked up to the next one closest in age, Holly, and would follow her everywhere she could get away with. Holly was kind and patient in her new role as a big sister after being the "baby" in the family prior to my new marriage.

    And now this news was hanging over his head.

Troy told me that if anything happened to him, he wanted me to be sure and tell Michelle, when she was old enough to understand, that this weekend together was planned way before we knew something was wrong. He wanted her to know that he wanted to spend time together, just the two of them.

Sweet Michelle, now you know. Your Papa loved you so much. But I think you've always known that.

While they were at the beach, I had a memorial service to go to. Mrs. Wiley had been a long time family friend and business associate, the wife of the late Stan Wiley. I had worked for Stan Wiley Realtors most of my real estate career. My oldest daughter, Summer, and ten-month-old Victoria went with me. Mrs. Wiley had been Summer's Sunday school teacher when we used to attend the Christian Science Church. That seemed like a lifetime ago.

After the service, we decided to take a walk through River View Cemetery. I had never been there before, or to any cemetery for that matter. Both of my parents had chosen to be cremated. There have been times when I wished there was an actual gravesite, a place to go and visit.

Something triggered in the back of my mind that this might be the cemetery where my brother was buried. My parents had never told me—they would never talk about it. I had not even known that I had an older brother until the sixth grade when my sister accidentally let it slip. He was only two years old when he died, just two weeks after I was born.

River View Cemetery is one of Portland's oldest and grandest cemeteries. We stopped at the office and inquired about anyone in the cemetery with the last name of LaBarre, my maiden name.

Yes! There were three by that name: my great Aunt Julia, a second name I didn't recognize, and my brother, Doug LaBarre.

We got a map, and after a lot of driving, sometimes in circles, we found the children's section of the cemetery. The grass was wet beneath our feet from the recent rain. Heavy gray clouds still hovered overhead, hiding the tops of the trees. I pulled Victoria closer to me, and wrapped her inside my raincoat to protect her from the cold, damp air. The graves were so small, so sad. There was no marker on Dougie's grave. Using the map, we walked down the rows until I found it next to a weeping cherry tree.

I was struck by the fact that Troy had given me a pair of this same kind of tree in memory of my mom and dad. Those trees were now planted side by side in our garden, and every spring they display a fresh garment of delicate pink blossoms.

Standing there with little Victoria in my arms, I finally had a chance to shed some tears for my brother whom I had never known. I think, though, that my tears were mostly for my mother. She carried her grief through her whole life. For a mother, losing a child is a sorrow beyond words.

§

Troy's mom was the first to notice it. She didn't say anything to us, but she was concerned. She detected a slight slur in her son's speech. Could he possibly have had a stroke? Or, as some at work had started to speculate, had Troy started drinking? A lot?

Now, as we waited for the test results, she agonized over whether she should say something. Sitting around the table at dinner the next weekend, Mom couldn't wait any longer. Not sure how to bring it up, she used humor as she and Troy were so accustomed to doing.

Jokingly she said, "Gee, Troy, how many beers did you have before dinner?"

Troy grew quiet, almost angry. "I didn't mean to offend you. I just noticed you were slurring your words a little," Mom said, wishing she had never said anything.

As a young girl, Marlene remembered seeing Lou Gehrig on a black and white newsreel in a theater. She remembered how deeply it affected her, thinking at the time that it had to be one of the worst things that could happen to a person.

The next day, May 8th, was Mother's Day. Three more days until the test results would be in. For Marlene, it was the worst Mother's Day of her life. She was in an agonizing wait. Waiting to hear what was wrong with her son, her only child. Waiting to hear, but not wanting to know.

"Oh Lord, please don't let it be that. Not Lou Gehrig's disease," was her constant prayer.

Troy was not just her only son — he was all the family she had. Marlene and her husband had divorced when Troy was eighteen. Her parents were gone, and what family she once had long ago disappeared.

Her mother had died shortly after giving birth to Marlene. Her father remarried, and it was not long before the stepmother made it clear she was not interested in raising three small girls. The girls were sent away to an orphanage.

The only one who seemed to truly care for these throw away children was a grandmother. Times were hard and money was in short supply, yet this "little old grandma" fought for those girls.

She became the role model for how Marlene would one day love her son and grandchildren. The girls made several trips in and out of orphanages before the grandmother was able to locate relatives who would take the girls. None of the families could take more than one child, so Marlene and her sisters were separated.

Marlene ended up across the country in Portland, Oregon, with an uncle. He and his wife were very poor. The aunt suffered from a severe mental disorder that made her constantly afraid that someone was trying to kill her. The uncle was an alcoholic.

It quickly became evident that the aunt had not agreed to do this out of the goodness of her heart. She used Marlene to do her work and take care of the house.

Because of her paranoia, she would make Marlene taste all of her food first in case it had been poisoned. She was convinced, for instance, that the milkman was going to poison the milk or that her husband was going to put something in her food to kill her.

Marlene's "bedroom" consisted of a sofa to sleep on and a nail on the wall to hang what few clothes she had. As a young girl, she would be sent to the taverns to fetch her uncle and bring him home when he was too drunk to find his way. She would have to walk alone in the dark in a seedy neighborhood, holding her breath the whole way there and back. She would be up late into the night, and then have to get up and go to school the next morning.

The fighting between her aunt and uncle was fierce. Yelling and screaming, the aunt would use Marlene as a shield to avoid the blows from her husband. More than once she was put in the middle as the uncle chased them with an ax.

"The poverty wasn't just a lack of money," Marlene recalls. "It was a home deprived of love and caring."

Oddly, Marlene was sent to church, although she would have to go by herself. Even though she had no choice in the matter, she was exposed to the missing ingredient in her childhood — love. It gave her something to hold on to.

Out of the dregs of this twisted childhood arose a spirit of determination in Marlene. She vowed she would never hurt anyone the way she had been hurt.

She dreamed of having a family some day. She dreamed of children and grandchildren of her own.

When her dream was realized and Troy was born, he could not have been more cherished. When he was a kid, he would go around singing, "I'm just a blessing in disguise," with a playful grin on his face. He had no idea how much of a blessing he truly was.

§

On Monday, the doctor's office called. The test results were back. When could we come in? The appointment was set for Wednesday, May 11th, at 2:00 p.m.

Troy said he didn't want me to go with him. I was shocked and hurt. Why was he pulling away when he needed me the most?

"I don't know what the news is going to be. If it's bad, I'm not sure what I'll do, how I will react. I don't want you to have to see that," he confessed. After some coaxing, and a few tears, he gave in and agreed to let me go with him.

Wednesday arrived. Troy hardly ever missed work and this day was no exception. He left the house at 5:30 a.m. as usual, and drove to Salem. Leaving work a couple hours early, he picked me up on the way to the doctor appointment.

"Maybe you should wait here," he said as we pulled into the parking lot. We were in downtown Portland at Good Samaritan Hospital. Troy had parked on the top level where there were fewer cars, plus it was outside. It was another beautiful sunny day. How could any news be too bad on a day like this?

"No way," I said. "Whatever the news is, we are in this together."

We rode the elevator down to the second floor. Troy knew where to go. He had been here less than two weeks before. He took my hand as we walked down two hallways to Dr. Gibbs' office.

"Please, have a seat," Dr. Gibbs gestured to the two chairs across from his desk.

Dr. Gibbs sat down at his desk. "We have gotten all the test results back. You don't have lead poisoning," he said.

That's a relief, I remember thinking.

"As a matter of fact, nothing really showed up on the tests. Why don't you come with me, and I'll show you the x-rays."

He led us down a long corridor to the lab. On the wall were x-rays of Troy's spinal column and brain.

"The good news is that there is nothing structurally wrong with your spine. Things look pretty normal," he explained.

We went back to his office and sat down again. Dr. Gibbs was being pleasant, almost too pleasant. He seemed nervous.

"The problem," he went on to say, "is that there is no real test that can be done for Amyotrophic Lateral Sclerosis, or as some call it, Lou Gehrig's disease. It is more a process of elimination. We start by ruling out all the other possibilities."

Troy was very quiet. His face was pale as he leaned forward in his chair, elbows on his knees. He stared at the floor without saying a word. We had learned enough by now to know that Amyotrophic Lateral Sclerosis is a rare neurological disease. There is no known cause…and no cure. And it is always fatal.

"So far, all the blood tests and x-rays have come back normal," he said, trying to sound positive. "I'm sending you to see Dr. Wendy Johnston at the Oregon Health Sciences University. She is the expert on ALS for the entire Northwest region. We're fortunate to have her here in Portland."

I was the first one to speak. "But Troy might not have this disease you're talking about, right? There is still a chance this could turn out to be nothing, isn't there?" I asked, my eyes pleading for an affirmative response.

"You'll have to wait and see what Dr. Johnston thinks," he replied hesitantly. This time I could see past the friendly face to a look of sympathy.

"But if she says you have the disease, you won't need to get any other opinions. I have already called ahead and told her about you. She is expecting to hear from you."

"And," Dr. Gibbs added, "I suggest you call and make an appointment as soon as possible."

At that, Troy quickly rose to his feet. He reached across the desk and shook Dr. Gibbs hand, thanking him for his time.

"Good luck," Dr. Gibbs said as we walked out of his office.

I was numb as we walked to the elevators. When we got to the truck, we sat there in silence, rolling down the windows to let out the late afternoon heat.

I waited for Troy to speak first, wanting to give my husband whatever space he needed.

When we finally looked at each other, Troy started chuckling. Then I started in. Before we knew it, we were both laughing uncontrollably. It was the weirdest thing I have ever experienced. We could not stop laughing. Tears were running down my face. A car pulled up next to us. The couple got out of the car and smiled at our laughter. They went away chuckling, too, wondering what could be so funny. Not in a million years would they have guessed where we had just come from.

The drive home was a blur. I don't remember anything about it until we pulled into the driveway. We were in shock — and I was in denial. I still refused to believe the worst. Fourteen-year-old Holly was home from school. When the phone rang, she answered it.

"It's for you, Mom," she said, bringing the phone outside to me.

Standing barefoot in the driveway, not even noticing how hot the pavement was getting under my feet, I took the phone. Troy had gone around back to work in the yard, his place of solace. It was Dr. Kilpatrick, the family doctor.

"Marilyn, I'm so very sorry," she said. "If there is anything I can do…"

"What do you mean?" I asked, frozen in my tracks. "Dr. Gibbs doesn't know yet what is wrong."

"He just didn't want to be the one to have to tell you," she replied. "He called me a few minutes ago. Marilyn…" she paused. "He would not be sending you to Dr. Johnston if he wasn't pretty sure that Troy has ALS."

Her words sent a shock wave through my body that felt like I had been struck by lightning. A cold chill ran through me despite the warm day. My breath caught in my throat and I couldn't speak. My mind flashed to an image of my father. A question had been tormenting me that I had not yet voiced, as I had tried so hard not to let myself think the unthinkable.

"Is ALS as bad as Parkinson's disease?" I managed to ask. My words were barely audible.

I remembered the nightmare of watching my dad suffer for five years until he died, as the muscles in his 6'4" body slowly betrayed him. I thought of my mother and what she went through caring for him.

"It's worse, Marilyn. Much worse…"

Reeling from the news, I hung up the phone and walked through the garage into the house, her last remarks about "living each day to its fullest" ringing in my head.

"Mom! What's wrong?" asked Holly, rushing over to me.

An anguished scream escaped from deep inside as I crumpled to the floor. Holly wrapped her arms around me and held me like a child as she waited to learn what was happening. Our whole world was crumbling around us…

§

The next thing I remember was one of the pastors from our church, Keith Reetz, at the front door. Troy had called him.

We joined Troy in the back yard and sat on the garden bench under the lace leaf maple. Troy had turned this corner of the backyard into a miniature Japanese garden. His potted bonsai plants framed the bench and gravel pathway. The late afternoon sun filtered down through the lacy leaves of the tree, making dancing shadows around our feet.

I will never forget the scripture Keith read to us that day, one that would be such a source of strength in the days ahead.

> "Fear not, for I have redeemed you; I have
> summoned you by name; you are mine. When
> you pass through the waters, I will be with you;
> and when you pass through the rivers, they will
> not sweep over you. When you walk through the
> fire, you will not be burned; the flames will not
> set you ablaze." (Isaiah 43:1-2)

After Pastor Keith left, Troy made the phone call to his mom. He asked her to come by when she got off work. When she arrived, they sat together in the living room. I stayed busy in the kitchen, wanting to give them space. This was a time for a mother and son to share alone.

When they walked back into the kitchen, Mom tried, like Dr. Gibbs, to be positive. She said something about how they would probably find a cure soon. She only stayed a few minutes, saying she needed to get home.

After everyone left, Troy and I were alone together with the suffocating realization that nothing would ever be the same. Sitting on his lap, I put my arms around his neck and we both sobbed inconsolably.

§

Marlene drove the half hour drive to her home in West Linn, trying to hold back the monstrous tidal wave that threatened to crash down on her at any moment. The house had never seemed so empty.

Unlocking the door, she went inside and sat down in the dark, waiting for the tears she knew would come when the shock wore off.

Sitting there in the silence of the darkness, unaware of how many hours had passed, the worst nightmare of her life started to sink in.

And the tears started to fall.

3
A DEATH SENTENCE

"If you are going through hell, keep going."
~Sir Winston Churchill (1874-1965)

Six days later, on May 17th, we walked into Dr.
Johnston's office at the Oregon Health and Sciences
University, a world class hospital and research center. Her
office, now turned into an ALS research center, was located on
the third floor in one of the older buildings. The elevator
smelled musty as it creaked and shuddered at each floor. The
hallways were painted turquoise and the paint was peeling at
the corners. The floors were large square tiles of flesh colored
linoleum with little black speckles.

As we walked into the small waiting area, a man in a
motorized wheel chair was just leaving. His head hung
forward, slightly tilted to one side. His hands lay limp in his
lap. His wrists and fingers were curled under from muscles
that would no longer cooperate. His wife had to operate the
wheelchair for him. In a voice that startled me as I stood there
trying not to stare, he slurred a 'good-bye' to the nurse.

No! This can't be! I thought as I tried to pull myself
together from what we had just seen. One look at my husband
told me he was thinking the same thing. A growing terror was

wrapping its tentacles around our throats, threatening to strangle both of us as we were put into an examination room to wait.

Dr. Johnston entered the room, apologizing for the wait. Quite a bit shorter than both of us, she wore glasses and had her blonde hair neatly tied back. Her slight accent depicted her Canadian roots. She was deeply kind as well as extremely knowledgeable. She asked several questions and tested Troy's reflexes. There were a couple more tests she wanted to order, mainly to rule out all other possibilities. (One of the tests was grueling for Troy. Using long needles, an electrical shock was sent into the muscles in his legs, arms and back to test reflex and strength.)

"But I have to tell you," she said. "I am pretty convinced that you have Amyotrophic Lateral Sclerosis." She paused before continuing. Looking into our faces she said, "This is the kind of diagnosis every doctor dreads giving a patient—and ALS is one of the most dreaded diseases."

She went on to explain that ALS is a motor neuron disease in which there is progressive death of the motor cells (neurons) in the brain and spinal cord. These motor cells control the muscles that enable us to move around, speak, breathe, and swallow. With no nerves to activate them, muscles gradually weaken and waste away. The progress is relentless and usually rapid. Almost cruelly, ALS leaves the mind intact. One has an active, healthy mind that becomes trapped in a motionless body. "It is like being on a desert island," she said.

Dr. Johnston asked about our family situation and history. No one else in Troy's family had ever had this disease which meant it wasn't the kind that is inherited. In about ten percent of cases, ALS is hereditary, referred to as familial ALS. Those families that have this "familial" type are tormented by this disease, which doesn't skip generations. A family that we learned of who live close by in Washington has already lost eight members to ALS with more showing symptoms.

When we told her that we had a baby daughter less than a year old, tears filled her eyes, and she cried with us. She, too, had a baby daughter.

"This is such a cruel disease, especially for someone as young as you," she said. We learned that the average age is around sixty years old. Troy was only 32.

"How long do I have?" Troy managed to ask. It was the only thing he had said in awhile.

"Usually anywhere from two to five years," she replied.

"But everyone is different," she quickly added. "No two cases are alike with this disease."

My first thought was that if Troy lived for five more years, Victoria would be in kindergarten when he died.

Dr. Johnston tactfully led the conversation to planning for the future. Troy could not handle it anymore. He had heard all he wanted to know for now. He left the room. I continued to ask questions. So many questions. The more I learned, the more I wished I had left the room when Troy did.

"No, there is no known cause. It's like a lightning strike," she explained. "It's just bad luck."

No, there was no cure. Not even any treatment at this time. We would mainly be focused on comfort care, she explained. She stressed the importance of starting to think about our living situation. Troy would probably be in a wheelchair within a year, possibly as soon as six months. Our house was two stories with all the bedrooms upstairs.

It was all so unbelievable! I kept thinking I was in some kind of a dream, a horrible nightmare. I kept trying to wake myself up to prove that this was not really happening.

Looking at Troy, you could never imagine that anything could be wrong with him. He looked so healthy and muscular! How could this tall, handsome, and healthy looking man be so sick? How could he have a disease we couldn't even pronounce?!

Two days later, we returned for the tests. We drove up the winding roads to the hospital in Troy's new convertible sports car, top down. The Oregon Health Sciences University sits on a hill overlooking the city of Portland. The house I grew up in was just up the hill from the hospital, and I had driven past it thousands of times. But this was the first time I had ever had reason to go there. Surrounded by tall fir trees, it is a maze of buildings spread out on the hillside with narrow, curvy roads winding around the different campuses. Nicknamed "Pill Hill," it can be a challenge finding your way around.

These winding roads were a jagged reminder of what our life had become. It was as if we had come to a sharp curve in the road and we couldn't see around the corner. The sign posted said "Stop, danger ahead!" We knew that somewhere around this next corner the road would come to the edge of a cliff. But we were powerless to stop. Our car was gaining speed and soon we would be unable to keep from plunging over the edge into a freefall.

That day, as we drove up the hill in the convertible, it started to rain. We didn't care. We did not even bother to put the top up. We just let the rain fall on us. Somehow, it seemed almost a comfort that this time the sun was not shining. The clouds seemed to understand and cry with us, as the rain soaked into our hair and clothes.

Troy smiled at me as he looked at my wet hair. He put in one of his favorite Van Morrison CDs:

Have I told you lately, that I love you?
Have I told you there's no one above you?
You fill my heart with gladness,
Take away the sadness.
Ease my troubles that's what you do.

At that moment, which is forever etched into my heart, I knew that whatever happened, we would get through it. I saw in Troy's eyes the strength and love I had come to depend on.

We were in this together…no matter what.

4
A RACE AGAINST TIME

"You can never learn that Christ is all you need,
until Christ is all you have."
~Corrie ten Boom

The days and weeks that followed seemed like they were on fast-forward. I desperately wanted to find the pause button. All I wanted to do was step outside of this life, even if only for a few weeks, and just hold Troy. Protect him. Keep him safe from this monstrous disease that took no prisoners, only casualties. Not knowing how much time we had sent us into a near panic mode trying to figure out how to spend whatever time we did have left.

I longed for someone to tell us what we should be doing. Should we take time off work? Travel? Should I quit my job and stay home for whatever time was left? I remembered a movie I had seen awhile back called "Lorenzo's Oil." In it, the mother and father devoted all their time and resources to find a cure for their son's incurable disease. Maybe we should be doing *that*...

I didn't want to miss a single precious minute with my husband. Yet, life doesn't stop, and we had a family to think about.

What do you do when your days are numbered? For Troy and I, there was only one clear thing we knew to do. Turn to the one who numbers our days. Turn to the God who holds us in his hands, and never lets us go.

§

The month of June was a crazy one for us, even in the best of circumstances. Three out of four daughters have birthdays in June. It is the end of the school year, and with our girls ranging in age from one to seventeen at the time, there was always some kind of graduation on the horizon. Throw in Father's Day in the same month, and there is not time for much else.

This particular June was Victoria's first birthday and Summer's graduation from Lake Oswego High School. All the activities that go along with graduation, including a big party at the house, were a good distraction. There were moments when my thoughts weren't absorbed with the dread and fear of what was ahead. But then the monster would always be lurking close by, threatening to come out and ruin the day.

Holly turned fifteen, which meant a trip to the DMV for her driver's permit. Now there's stress—a second teenage driver in the house! By that point, Summer had three "learning experiences" to her name. The first time she crunched the driver's door of the Jeep at Dairy Queen. Next, she backed into the neighbor as he was coming out of his driveway. The third, and probably most notable (not to mention expensive!), was when she ran into a Mercedes at a four way stop while driving Troy's car.

For Victoria's first birthday, we had a small family party at home. Bert and Susy Waugh, Victoria's godparents, joined us along with their three teenage boys. We all tried to carry on as normally as possible, joking around and making small talk.

Several times, I observed Troy standing off to the side by himself. I watched as he looked at his precious little daughter. He was struggling to maintain his composure, and I knew he was thinking about the years ahead that he would be missing.

Then Troy's dad came for a visit from Arizona for Father's Day. Our time was not our own. I so badly wanted to hit a pause button. To slow things down in this unknown amount of time we had left. Instead, we were being swept along like a toy boat on a white water river.

For the fourth of July, we took the family to the beach house. I looked around the house that we had bought together, furnished together, wall-papered together. So many good memories, but so many more that could have been, that should have been. The thought of taking care of it by myself, of being alone here, terrified me.

After finally getting through all the family obligations, it was our turn. The next week Troy and I took a trip, just the two of us. We were desperate to try to get in whatever time and memories we could before it was too late.

We drove the sports car to Canada for the weekend. The time was so bittersweet. Knowing that this time spent together was one of endings rather than beginnings, that our life together would soon be in the past, was almost more than I could bear.

I wrestled with my thoughts, trying to stay strong and keep positive, grasping at how to navigate the overwhelming emotions. Savoring the moment didn't work — the happier the moments, the sadder they were for me. Instead, I would try hard to sketch each moment into my mind, to carve it on my heart so at least I would have memories to savor after he was gone. All I could do was store away the memories so they would be there to pull off the shelf in the times to come when I would be alone.

One of those moments I was able to "sketch" into my memory was on the drive up. After heading north on I-5, we turned off onto Hwy 101 and headed west toward Port Angeles. The drive is beautiful as the road follows the Hood Canal much of the way. With the sparkling water to the right, the tall fir trees give flashes of shade as the car races along. The top is down on our sports car, and the wind is warm as I feel it whipping through my hair. We are listening to one of our favorite artists, Van Morrison, singing:

"I look at the side of your face
As the sunlight comes
Streaming through the window…
I'm thinking wouldn't it be great?
If it was like this all the time."

It was one of the rare moments where I was able to find the pause button, and for just a few minutes, I could enjoy the moment, filled with the joy of being together on this adventure, looking over at Troy driving with a smile on his face.

We arrived at the docks in Port Angeles, Washington, around 5:00 p.m. It was Friday afternoon and everyone wanted to get somewhere for the weekend. We barely made it on the last ferry for the evening. Even though by now it was close to 7:30 p.m., it was still warm outside, and the cool breeze off the water felt good. At this time of year in the Northwest, it doesn't get dark until close to 10:00 p.m., so the sun had barely started its descent toward the horizon.

When we arrived on the Canadian side, the customs officials boarded the boat. There were several rows of cars funneling through the gates to the dock. A uniformed agent motioned us to get out of the line.

Two agents came over to our car and told us to pull off to the side and get out. Everyone in the cars around us were staring or pointing as we parked the convertible and got out. We were told to wait there.

Not only was it embarrassing, I was getting irritated at the delay. We were already a couple of hours behind schedule because of the long lines at the ferry. Now this.

A woman in a uniform told Troy to open the trunk and glove box. She took my purse and emptied it out onto the seat. The next thing I knew she and another agent wheeled a metal cart over and started pulling our luggage out.

"Now wait just a minute! What is going on here?" I demanded.

The woman shot me a look of warning, and told me to step back against the wall. Troy took my arm and pulled me back next to him. I asked him what was going on.

"Don't say anything," he said in a low voice. "Just do what they ask, and we'll get out of here a lot quicker."

The two agents disappeared for several minutes. When they came back, they opened our suitcases and started taking everything out and putting it on the metal cart. I could hardly contain myself!

All the anger that had been building over the past several weeks — stemming from the helplessness of not being able to stop the disease, and the knowledge of how the short time we had left together that was evaporating before our eyes — all came flooding to the surface. This customs agent was about to have a wall of fury unleashed on her.

Troy could sense it coming and put his arm tightly around my waist.

"Don't do it," he warned. "I don't want to spend our weekend together in jail."

The woman walked over to us, and with no explanation, she said we could leave now. Not even an, "I'm sorry for the inconvenience!" Didn't even put our stuff back into the suitcases. We never knew what it was they were looking for or why we appeared so suspicious. Maybe it was the red sports car. Whatever it was, I realized that day how much anger and frustration had built up inside of me.

Troy's turn was next. We drove down wide tree-lined streets through a neighborhood of old European style homes with stunning yards and gardens. When we arrived at the beautiful Bed and Breakfast Inn where we were staying, he went to get our luggage. As he tried to juggle the bags, he dropped one. I went to pick it up and he snapped at me that he could get it. He wanted to carry them all, even though his strength was already deteriorating. He had always been that way. No matter how many bags of groceries we had, he would carry all of them. It wasn't that I was not capable — but his chivalry was one of the many things I loved about him. It was painful to watch him try to juggle the luggage, his arms not cooperating. The frustration and anger was beginning to overtake him, too.

That night we knelt together in prayer. I'll never forget Troy's prayer. He didn't ask God to take away the disease. What he prayed for was the courage and strength to face it — however hard it got.

§

I had been so hopeful that this little get-away would give him rest, and maybe renew his strength. I wanted to believe that it was because I usually saw him at the end of a long day of work that he was looking so tired. It soon became apparent that was not the case.

Being with him twenty-four hours a day, I could actually see things change. His speech was starting to slur more and more. The deep, sexy voice that I loved so much was starting to crack, like a teenage boy going through puberty. There were times when his blue eyes would become dull, almost glazed over, as his body fought the disease.

It was very frightening to me not to be able to tell what he was thinking as his facial features and body language started to change. At times, it was almost like being with a stranger. I was trying to get to know him all over again, to read his thoughts as I was accustomed to doing, trying to understand what he was going through.

It was becoming more and more difficult to read his body language, to learn his limitations, to figure out how to communicate, to understand his changing humor as his speech became more limited and difficult. And it was always changing. Weekly. Daily. The loneliness threatened to overwhelm me, even when I was with him.

I watched him go through the physical pain from his deteriorating muscles. But the pain of processing what was happening was a far deeper pain. I watched as he became more withdrawn, off in a different place with his thoughts as he struggled to cope with the disease.

It was in these times of helplessness and fear that I would cry out to God, my shelter in the storm.

It was there that I would find the strength to go on. It was there that I would find the courage to face the future.

It was there that I would hang on to his promise that he gives us the gift of his grace to cover whatever the need is. One day at a time.

"Let us then approach the throne of grace with confidence, so that we may receive mercy and find grace to help us in our time of need." (Hebrews 4:16)

In time, I would learn all over again how to "read" my husband's thoughts. We would come to know a completely new level of communication.

§

A big decision we faced was what to do about our house. Just a month before we found out about Troy's illness, we had purchased a piece of property in the Yamhill wine country. Our dream was to have a small acreage property with a view, to raise nursery stock for Troy's future landscaping business, and to build our dream house.

We found the perfect spot in the hills of Newberg, a small town twenty miles west of Portland. The 180-degree view was breathtaking, overlooking vineyards and the town of Newberg. You could see for miles. Our plan had been to build in three years when Holly graduated from high school.

Dr. Johnston advised that if we decided to go ahead and build the house, we had better do it soon. The disease was progressing at an alarming rate, surprising even her.

We knew we couldn't stay in the house we were in with all the bedrooms and showers on the second floor. But most friends advised against building, thinking it would be too stressful to take on such an undertaking at this point.

We were in a quandary on what to do, but after much prayer decided to go ahead with the new house. It made sense that we could design a house that would be wheelchair accessible. For us, it proved to be a good diversion from the merciless progression of the disease.

We found it hard even to have a conversation that did not center on the disease. We would go out to dinner together and try to make a pact not to talk about the illness. Most of the time, we were unsuccessful.

By going ahead with our dream, we had something to look forward to. Something to plan together. Something we could watch being built, instead of torn down and destroyed.

By August, we had our house ready to go on the market. In-between the increasing procession of doctor appointments, physical therapists, speech therapists, naturopathic treatments, etc. were meetings with builders and suppliers. Every time we met with a medical professional, it was a discouraging reality checkpoint. Every meeting with the builder was a welcome diversion.

We received an offer on our house in September. We found an apartment close by that would keep Holly in the same school district. Things were falling into place. But the night before we were to put down the deposit on an apartment we got word that the sale on our house had failed.

Our plans unraveled. We were in limbo again, wondering if we should go ahead with the building plans. Our spirits and our tempers were wearing thin. The pressure was putting a strain on our family. We were getting irritable and frustrated. And tired — always so very tired.

Almost every night I cried myself to sleep, most of the time waiting until after Troy had fallen asleep. It was when the house was finally quiet and I was alone with my thoughts that I could not control the tears and sadness. Many nights I would wake up in the middle of the night, and the tears would start all over again.

It was during these darkest hours that I would have heart-to-heart talks with God. He reminded me of the ways he had met my needs in the past. After my dad died, he brought me Bert and Pastor Ron (both 6'4" like my Dad, by the way). Troy came into my life and was there for me when my mom died three years later.

With our marriage came a new mom, Marlene. Not that we can ever replace a loved one, but in his timing, God fills the emptiness that is left with new love.

When it came to losing Troy, however, it was unthinkable. I argued with God on this one. I didn't want a new husband!

In a very tender and emotional moment, Troy told me that after he was gone he wanted me to marry again. He wanted that for Victoria, too. He wanted her to have a father around as she was growing up. I felt as if I had just been stabbed in the heart with a knife. I knew he was saying it totally out of unconditional love. I could only imagine how incredibly difficult it was for him to say that. But the very thought of anyone else but Troy was unbearable. I made a silent vow, right or wrong, to raise her by myself and devote all my time and emotional energy to her.

Just three months after the diagnosis, Troy's condition was already deteriorating at an alarming rate. The twitching, a sign that a muscle was dying, seemed to be happening at different places all over his body. His ability to write was almost gone; his neck muscles were getting weaker; and his arms had grown too weak even to put his coat on by himself. His shoulders were starting to slouch forward when he walked.

In the morning, I would follow him to the garage, take his keys and find the right key to his car. He had very little strength left in his hands so I would put the key in what grip his fingers had left. He needed me to open the car door. He was able to do it from the inside, but not the outside.

I wondered if he left his coat on all day at work and didn't close the car door when no one was around to help him. I would pray the whole time he was driving, knowing that he already was past the point where it was really safe. Giving up driving had to be one of the toughest things for him. He had always loved cars, and it was one of the greatest losses of his independence when he had to stop driving.

The day he came home with a dent in the front fender of the sports car from a run-in with a pickup truck was the day he knew it was over. It was the kind of accident that he would normally have been able to avoid, if his body had reacted as fast as his mind did. I was just thankful he finally admitted it before anything more serious happened.

Dr. Johnston was starting to question us on how long it would take to build the house. Wondering what her concern was, I asked the question. She confided that due to the rapid deterioration Troy was experiencing, it appeared that he might have only a year left…or less. We were in shock all over again! What had happened to three to five years? What about Victoria's kindergarten???

We learned that there are two different types of ALS onset. If the symptoms and decline start in the lower body, it is because the neurons in the spine are the first to start dying. If it starts in the upper body, usually affecting speech and swallowing early on, it is called "bulbar onset." In this case, the neurons in the brain are the first to be affected.

This is the kind that Troy apparently had. The prognosis from the start of symptoms to death is much quicker, as the weakness reaches the lungs faster. Our nightmare was getting worse.

"Can you get the house built in nine months?" Dr. Johnston asked me privately. We were used to having Troy leave the room as soon as possible.

"If not, I doubt that Troy will ever live there."

§

When we left the doctor's office that day, we decided to take a drive out to the property.

It was a glorious fall day. Late September in Oregon is one of the most beautiful times of the year. The days are usually sunny and warm, and the nights cool way down as nature prepares for winter. The leaves were changing into their autumn colors of auburn and crimson. The hillside vineyards were turning into rows of gold. The smell of wood burning stoves hung in the air. Looking out from the property, we could see a mist in the valley that wove in and out of the tops of the fir trees like a white ribbon. The sun was just starting to set, casting long shadows across the hills. At the same time, the moon was already starting its journey upward into the northern sky.

Holding hands, we knelt down on our property. Looking out across the valley, we asked God to show us what he would have us do with the land.

Driving home at dusk, with the top still down on the car and the chilly evening air blowing against our face, we made the decision to move ahead with building the house.

The sale fail on our Lake Oswego house turned out to be a blessing. In the interim, we found a different apartment, this time a three bedroom, one-story apartment that was on the ground level. As soon as we found it, the sale came back to life on our house.

In retrospect, had we moved into the first apartment, we wouldn't have been able to stay there because of the two levels.

During the ten months it took to build the house, Troy would decline to the point where there was no way we could have managed stairs. It was another testimony of God's care for us, letting us know we were not walking through this alone.

5
HELPING HANDS, SEEN AND UNSEEN

"Only in the darkness, you are able to see the stars."
~Martin Luther King

One evening in October, three weeks before we moved out of our house, I was making dinner and Troy was playing with Victoria. It was our usual routine these days after he came home from work. Troy, tired from working all day, would shower and change into a pair of his favorite faded Levis. Coming downstairs, he would find Victoria so they could play.

Troy's job with the county was such a physically demanding one that we knew changes would have to be made before long.

By September, he cut back to working four days a week. On Mondays, he stayed home with Victoria. It was such a special time for the two of them, one that he cherished.

Over the summer, Victoria had transitioned from baby to toddler. She had entered that wonderful time of discovery of the world—her first words, her first steps. She liked to pull the clothes out of the laundry basket. She would drag Troy's shirt around the house, saying "papa" over and over. Whenever she said his name, she would make kissing sounds.

At mealtime, she now wanted to try to feed herself. She put the food on the spoon, but most of the time it wouldn't stay on all the way to her open mouth. Troy was having the same difficulty.

Victoria was becoming more independent, learning to say more words, learning how to walk and run. At the same time, her dad was learning how to be dependent on others, to say fewer words, to slow down his physical activity. The symbolism was striking. As Troy's life on this earth was draining away, it was being deposited into this "unexpected" blessing of a daughter. Beyond anything Troy could have planned or orchestrated, his legacy was being carefully written and preserved in this next generation.

As I was making dinner that evening, I could hear Victoria squealing with delight as her papa "chased" her around the living room. Since she hadn't perfected walking yet, she was much faster at crawling.

Troy used to crawl after her during this game, but when his arms couldn't support him any longer he would just bend over and chase her. They came around the corner into the kitchen where I was cooking dinner at the stove.

Just as I turned my head to look over at them, Troy lost his balance. He was toppling forward, right on top of little Victoria!

In that split second, as I watched helpless to stop him, he fell face first onto the hardwood floor. He knew that his arms were useless to catch him, and if he landed on his chest he would have crushed Victoria underneath him.

Instead, he used his face to break the fall of his 200-pound body.

"Holly, help me!" I screamed.

Holly came running down the stairs from her bedroom. It was the place she spent most of her time these days. My heart aches when I think of how little time I had available for Holly, my daughter who didn't demand it the way some kids do. She instead tried to please people, and was our happy go lucky, fun loving and free spirited child. These days, with our world upside down, she stayed away from the stress and chaos and kept to herself. She was left to navigate the early teenage years mostly on her own. With a new marriage, a new child, and now this illness, her mom was no longer available. Her way of dealing with the nightmare we were living was to quietly withdraw.

I rolled Troy over as Holly grabbed the crying Victoria. Blood trickled down from a deep cut on his forehead, and his nose was smashed and starting to swell. In a panic, he was making loud moaning sounds, unable to verbalize in words.

Kneeling beside him, I told him, "it's going to be okay, it's going to be okay." But I wasn't so sure. Then I realized that his concern was for Victoria. He was trying to tell me to go to her instead of trying to help him.

Holly had taken her into the living room, away from the frightening scene of Troy's bleeding face. She was holding her and rocking her, but could not get her to stop crying.

"Bring Victoria here," I yelled.

When Holly brought her into the kitchen, her crying stopped. I took her from Holly, but she squirmed and wanted down. As soon as I put her down on the floor, she went right over to her papa and started gently patting his shoulder, saying "papa, papa" and making kissing sounds. She had been as concerned about him as he was about her.

Holly helped me get them into the Suburban and we headed for the hospital. I was shaking uncontrollably as I called his mom on the cell phone, asking her to meet us at emergency.

Miraculously, Victoria checked out fine with just a bump to her forehead. There had been some unseen arms of protection around her that night.

Troy's nose was broken, but the cuts on his face didn't require stitches. And in typical Troy fashion, he asked me to pray with him for the man in the bed next to him.

§

Three weeks later, with the help of ten of Troy's co-workers (not the inmates!) we moved into the apartment. We were so thankful that a loving heavenly Father was constantly watching over us and made sure that we had not moved into the original upper unit apartment. Troy was already having difficulty with stairs.

Troy had cut back to three days a week, and was starting to do a design project on the computer. His supervisors were awesome about finding ways he could stay employed with his increasing levels of disability. It was very important to him to keep working for as long as possible, to feel useful and maintain whatever part of a "normal" life he could.

Troy made the difficult decision that he could no longer take care of Victoria on Mondays. He really hated to give that up. But he was getting concerned about safety and his ability to take care of her if something happened.

Our plan was to spend Thanksgiving at the beach house. We didn't know how many more times we would be able to go as a family. Troy announced that he wanted to drive down by himself a day ahead of us. I didn't like the idea one bit, but he seemed to really want the independence and solitude. Who could blame him? It would probably be his last chance. He drove the sports car, and did okay on the drive down. He called several times and reassured me he was doing okay.

Unfortunately, he fell that night getting into bed. He didn't break anything this time, but he scraped his back up pretty bad. Falling is common with ALS as balance becomes a problem, in addition to the weakness.

One time at the apartment, Troy had gone into Holly's room to get one of his CDs that she had borrowed. Apparently when he leaned over to get it off the shelf, he fell. He yelled for me and I came running to see what was wrong. I found him on his side, with his upper body wedged between the bed and the tall shelves.

"What on earth happened?" I asked, amused. "How did you do that? What were you trying to get?"

"Just get me out of here!" he exclaimed.

§

January 5th was Troy's last day of driving. It was around this time that a good friend of ours, Mike Sawyer, offered to come over once a week and spend time with Troy — to be his arms and hands. It was such a relief and encouragement to me, knowing that someone else was willing to commit to share the burden. Not just saying, "let me know if there is anything I can do to help," but actually suggesting a way that he could offer tangible support.

They would take rides in the convertible, and work on designing a fountain Troy wanted for the front courtyard of the new house.

We tried leaving Victoria with them when Mike was there to help. But it tore Troy up inside to see another man able to pick up his daughter, and do the things he longed to do. He grieved for hours after, and we decided it was not worth the anguish it caused him and arranged for other help with Victoria.

Mike continued to faithfully come and keep Troy company. They would have long talks, and Mike asked Troy if he would put on paper what he was learning during this time when he knew he did not have much time left. Out of this came what Troy and Mike, in jest, called "The Manly List."[1]

With the help of my brother, Larry, and his computer expertise, Troy got set up with an AutoCAD program to do landscape design work. It was a way he could still contribute as an employee. As Troy's hands became increasingly useless, he found a different way to adapt to the computer. He started operating the mouse with his foot. It was slow going, but Troy persevered.

Our oldest daughter, Summer, was now a Freshman at George Fox University in Newberg. She helped out as much as she could in between schoolwork and campus life, coming over every Thursday to the apartment to run errands and do housework. It hadn't been that long ago that Summer had been quite upset at my announcement that I was getting married. Understandably, she wasn't excited that our life was about to change. It had been just the three of us for as long as she could remember. Then there wasn't much time to adjust to having a step-dad in the house before Victoria came along. But thankfully, Summer was excited about the new addition and it was a turning point in her attitude towards this new blended family. She was a big help with Victoria and really stepped up to the plate with a changed heart towards Troy when the diagnosis came.

I was so thankful she chose a college close by. She and her boyfriend, Greg, would come on the weekends when they could. We tried our best to continue life, enjoying family time and making memories. I can still picture Greg sprawled out on our living room floor reading the Sunday paper with Victoria climbing all over him. We even managed to make it to one of Greg's soccer games when George Fox was playing nearby. Summer and I maneuvered Troy's wheelchair next to the bleachers with Victoria on his lap. It was always so great

---

[1] See Appendix, "Manly List"

to do something "normal," even if we did make quite a spectacle.

The support of friends and family was a beacon of light in a stormy sea. Pastor Keith from church came by regularly and visited with Troy. Holly ran errands with her new driver's license. Marlene came every weekend and took care of Victoria so I could tend to Troy's needs.

One evening we received an unexpected call. It was a woman who had lost her husband to this same horrible disease just three weeks earlier. She offered us the use of some of the equipment that had belonged to her husband, including a virtually new laptop computer with software for a special mouse and on-screen keyboard. From the first time we met her, Mary Beth Baker became a wonderful friend, and a huge support. Her infectious laugh and fun sense of humor could always make Troy smile, and in spite of her recent loss and enormous grief, she visited often. Between the two of them, we would all be in stitches during her visits, which were a welcome medicine.

Troy enjoyed showing people his landscape drawings on the new computer. He was showing some to Mary Beth one day, and then showed her a stick figure that he had drawn.

"What the heck is that?" she asked.

He told her it was his new signature since he could no longer type his name.

"It does kind of look like you these days," she teased.

§

Now that Troy was no longer driving, I took him to Salem once a week to meet with an architect at his work and go over his project. Just getting ready was beginning to take up most of the morning.

I would help him shower, although getting in and out of a tub shower was getting increasingly difficult and dangerous. He needed me to put on his shirts because he couldn't pull them over his head anymore, and buttons were difficult. Socks were also a chore. His hands couldn't grab things.

And then there was the shaving thing. Oh my gosh, was that ever a test of our marriage! He was so picky on how it should be done! I never seemed to go the right direction with the razor, or else I would accidentally cut him. It took so long, I think his beard started to grow back before I finished.

When it came to brushing teeth, we figured out a way that I would support his arm at the elbow. Then using an electric toothbrush he could manage to do most of it himself.

But all these things we figured out and adapted to would change within weeks, sometimes even days. ALS is a disease that requires constant adaptation. It seemed like as soon as we figured out a solution, his condition would deteriorate and we would have to come up with something new.

On one of these trips back from Salem, we stopped at a fast food restaurant and picked up hamburgers. Driving with one hand, I was feeding Troy with the other. He could drink from a straw, but needed me to hold the cup. Trying to feed him a hamburger, and keep my eyes on the road at the same time was a real challenge. Ketchup would be dripping all over the place, or I would look away at the wrong time and miss his mouth, smashing the hamburger into the side of his face instead.

It was too late by the time I noticed the state trooper on the side of the highway. I hadn't paid close enough attention to the speedometer (how many things can a person do at one time?), and here came the patrol car, lights flashing.

I pulled the suburban over, and turned off the motor. I quickly tried to wipe the mustard off my hands as I rolled down the window.

"May I see your license, please?" he asked. "Did you know that you were going fifteen miles an hour over the speed limit, ma'am?"

"Well, actually, no I didn't," I replied. "But it was because my husband was distracting me."

"Your husband was distracting you," he repeated, mockingly. Eyebrows raised, he looked past me into the car at Troy.

"Well, I mean, it's not what it sounds like," I said, now totally flustered. I explained to him about Troy's illness and how I had been trying to feed him. The officer softened, and let me off the hook without a ticket.

"But please, try and be more careful next time," he warned.

§

On January 16th, we broke ground on the new house. I drove Troy out there to watch as the bulldozers started moving dirt to carve out the footprint of the house.

There were so many mixed emotions for Troy. It was exciting to see; yet he was very discouraged at not being able to do the landscaping he had been so looking forward to.

At this point, though, our biggest hope was that Troy would live long enough to see the house finished. There was growing concern that he wouldn't make it that long.

I was carrying such a huge load. Besides working full time to support the family, there were the growing number of medical appointments to arrange, usually several a week. Besides the neurologist, there was physical therapy, occupational therapy, pulmonologist (lung specialist), speech therapist, and then some more we added ourselves like the naturopath and acupuncturist.

I was extremely thankful that my boss, Bert, was so understanding and supportive. He let me take Wednesdays off and work a four-day week. Building a house is a maze of decisions, inspections, and meetings. Thank God for my organizational skills. But I fear that I was a builder's worst nightmare. The tremendous pressure we felt to get the house built as quickly as possible was put onto our poor builder.

Building on a hillside in the middle of winter in Oregon is slow going at best. Before we even broke ground, the well had to be dug. After three days, they had drilled down 450 feet and finally hit water, eight gallons per minute.

But Troy wasn't satisfied. He knew this was minimal for a household, let alone irrigating over two acres of landscaping. He told them to keep going. Just past 525 feet, they broke through the bedrock and hit water at thirty-five gallons per minute. We were ecstatic!

Next, a road had to be built up to the building site. Troy knew just how he wanted the long driveway to be. It was amazing how he had such a keen eye for design and could see it in his mind. He had always been good at design, as an amateur black and white photographer.

I observed that as the disability progressed and his physical strength waned, his other faculties sharpened. He became amazingly observant. Whenever I would forget where I had put something, which was becoming quite commonplace (extreme stress plays havoc with your memory!), I would ask Troy. He didn't miss a thing!

With the AutoCAD program on the computer, he was able to draw the driveway just how he wanted it. At first, the builder and the heavy equipment operators didn't get it. They couldn't picture it, and wanted to just make a straight line with a switchback.

But Troy did not back down. With a long rectangle to work with, he used the 250+ foot driveway to divide the property into pleasing shapes.

After a gentle curve at the bottom, the driveway switched back into a long sweeping curve. At the top, above the house, it split into a circular drive around a hundred year old, magnificent black walnut tree.

Even the builder was amazed at how well it turned out.

Inside the long curve was to be a huge, sweeping lawn. Lining the driveway, he wanted flowering cherry trees. We were so touched when four of his co-workers arrived in pickups pulling trailers, loaded with flowering cherry trees. Before the day was over, they had them all planted, just the way Troy had envisioned.

For our anniversary that year, my forever-romantic husband gave me a "Rose Garden." He had ordered seventy-five old English rose bushes! His co-worker, Guy, who had helped plant the trees, brought up a cat and cleared a large rectangle above the circular drive. With Troy's instructions, he planted a stunning, old-fashioned rose garden.

And as it turned out, the place Troy ordered the roses from refused to accept payment. They had been one of the suppliers that Troy worked with at the county. It was a way they could help.

These acts of kindness, and the incredible love and support we felt, helped to keep us going. We came to learn and experience firsthand that God truly balances the scales. The tougher things get on the one side, the more the blessings are poured out on the other.

6
A LIVING MEMORIAL

"In the end, it's not the years in your life that count.
It's the life in your years."
~Abraham Lincoln

It was Valentine's Day and the snow had been falling steadily since the night before. There was a good foot of snow (well, maybe it was only four or five inches) accumulated on the ground outside the apartment. I love the way the snow makes everything so quiet—just the occasional car spinning its tires trying to make it up the hill. It was Wednesday, my day off, and Troy and I were going to get to spend the day together. No doctor appointments. No having to rush off to work.

I had just gotten out of the shower. Standing in the bathroom in a white terry cloth robe, I was drying my hair.

When I turned off the hair dryer, I heard a blood chilling sound. It sounded almost animal-like, a kind of moaning.

It took just a split second to realize that the sound coming from the living room was Troy. I raced down the hall to the living room. He was lying on the floor on his side, a large red bloodstain forming on the carpet underneath his head. I was horrified to think how long he might have been lying there while I had been unable to hear him. The blood was coming from his nose, which was literally pushed sideways on his face. More blood was on the side of an upholstered armchair that he had hit on his way down. He was unable to tell me what had happened, but I learned later that he had lost his balance and fallen. His arms were useless to stop the fall, and his face hit the hard arm of the chair on the way down. That was what broke his nose — again.

"Oh my God, honey, I am so sorry. I am so sorry," was all I could say. I grabbed the phone and dialed 911. I was afraid to move him. By now, the moaning sounds had stopped. He lay very still and I was afraid he was going into shock. His breathing was shallow, and his eyes were starting to glaze over.

The paramedics arrived quickly in spite of the snow. After a brief recount of what had happened and Troy's medical condition, they loaded him onto a stretcher. There was not time for me to get ready and go with them. Standing in my bathrobe, I watched them wheel my husband down the sidewalk through the snow.

"I'll be right behind you, honey. Don't worry, it's going to be okay," I called after them.

I closed the door against the cold air that had been rushing into the warm apartment. Leaning back against the door, I looked at the large red bloodstain on the carpet.

"How much more can he take?" I shouted in anger to an empty room. Hot tears were streaming down my cheeks. But there was no time for crying or anger. I had to get to the hospital. My husband needed me.

§

This second broken nose required immediate surgery. No options this time. After getting through the whole nightmare of the fall and the surgery, we got a medic-alert call system. It was a speakerphone with a remote control that hung around Troy's neck. If he pushed the button, the phone would automatically turn on. If no phone number was entered within a few seconds, the phone would automatically speed dial whatever number you programmed in. For us, it was 911.

I could not help but notice that the second number on the speed dial was not my work number. It was Captain Video, Troy's favorite movie and surround sound video systems store!

In April, we had a second pulmonary test done, to measure Troy's breathing capacity. This is the critical issue with ALS. His pulmonologist, Dr. Edwards, met with us in his office to discuss the results.

"Based on the rate of progression of respiratory muscle decline since your last test, it appears that you have up to six months before you will require full time ventilation," Dr. Edwards said. "Of course, this will be sooner if there are complications such as at-risk pneumonia."

In other words, unless Troy agreed to go on a ventilator, he had possibly six more months left to live. Actually, we came away from that appointment encouraged. A quick mental calculation told me that if the builder finished the house in May or June as expected, Troy would get to live there—at least for a few months.

By April, Troy had to give up working. Even the computer work was becoming too draining. Conserving energy just for the daily tasks of living became a priority. His weight was now down to165 pounds, a loss of 75 pounds in less than a year.

The staff at the county had been planning a memorial for him. They wanted him to see it while he was still able. It had been kept a secret from Troy until now.

In the Japanese garden, in an inner courtyard surrounded by the staff offices, they were building a pond in honor of Troy. It was so fitting that they chose the Japanese garden. Troy had designed and maintained it, and it was one of his favorite spots. In the past, when I could manage the time to come visit him for lunch, we would usually sit out there.

The pond was finished and the day of the dedication arrived. We decided it was best at that point to tell him what was going on. In his fragile condition, I didn't think a big surprise would have been a good idea.

As we drove to Salem, I could tell he was nervous. I can only imagine what it must have been like for him, what thoughts were going through his head.

He was on his way to see his own memorial.

How many of us will ever experience that?

For that matter, how many of us would ever receive a memorial?

We arrived around noon. Troy was wearing a dark blue sports coat and blue and white striped dress shirt. A little different from how they were used to seeing him dressed!

I pushed Troy in his portable wheelchair to the front door of the main entrance. He could still walk, slowly, but we wanted to conserve his energy for this big event. Marlene and Victoria also went with us. It was a breezy day, with an occasional sun break in the clouds. By the time we got outside in the courtyard, a light rain had started. The wind was whipping through the pointed green leaves of the tall bamboo.

The courtyard was packed with people. Some were supervisors, or officers in uniform. Some were office staff, shivering under umbrellas. Then there were the guys who Troy worked with on a daily basis on the landscape maintenance. Two of the guys, Bobby and Guy, one on each side, helped Troy up the two steps to see the pond. It was designed in the Japanese motif with bamboo troughs for the water to spill down, and Koi fish in the pond. There was a plaque honoring Troy and his dedication to his work.

Crowded around the perimeter, with either a coffee cup or cigarette in one hand, many seemed self-conscious or uncomfortable with how to handle this unusual occasion.

"Is this a line-up?" one of the officers joked. As we stood and admired the fountain, a few at a time would come up and speak to Troy.

Everyone was trying to keep it light-hearted, but I noticed several that had to turn their heads to hide the tears.

Victoria offered the much-needed distraction, as she did so often. She stole the show with her cute antics and joy, oblivious to the profound sadness of this event. Troy looked at her so tenderly, so proud, as many admired what a doll his daughter was.

We moved indoors to a large visiting room, lined with orange plastic chairs. Taking a deep breath, Ted Nelson, the jail commander (head honcho!), introduced a few people who wanted to speak. Troy was seated in his wheelchair in the front row. Cameras were flashing from different parts of the room.

We were surprised when Mick was the first to speak. He was wearing one of those long, dark brown Australian oilskin raincoats over his Levis and blue county shirt. On his head was a wide-brimmed leather stockman hat, his long ponytail hanging down his back. He had one hand in his pocket and a white Styrofoam coffee cup in the other. He leaned back against the counter, trying to be casual to hide his nervousness.

"When I first come out here," he started, "everyone knew I didn't have the greatest reputation and stuff. It was Troy's communication, not so much the words, but the attitude...well, it was very inspirational. Actually, it humiliated me quite a bit. Didn't refrain completely, but I toned down my gestures and comments and stuff." He paused, trying to keep his emotions in check.

"I think I've become a better person," Mick continued, choosing his words carefully. "It was like a tough love thing that Troy threw at me. It wasn't the easiest thing for him to see. Would have been a lot easier to ignore me. But rather than ignore me, he took the time and told me how he saw it. I respect that. And I'm better for it."

With tears in his eyes, and voice wavering, he said, "and I thank you very much, from the bottom of my heart.

Bob, Troy's supervisor, was the next to speak. He presented a plaque and read these words written on it:

DEDICATED TO TROY THOMPSON
All of your friends at Marion County would like to thank you for all that you have given to us!
There's nothing that you would not do for us. You are always there, willing to help, no task too big. Your positive, up-beat attitude always brightens our days.
We know that you love the outdoors and gardening, because you have taken great pride and care in the landscaping for Marion County.
We dedicate to you, with love and appreciation, the pond in the Japanese Garden.
Your friends at Marion County

With that, Bob walked over and put the plaque in Troy's lap. He put his arms around him and gave him a big hug.

That's when Troy lost it. The tears were unstoppable. By now, I don't think there was a dry eye in the place.

Ted came over, and put a hand on Troy's shoulder. Knowing how difficult and emotional this was getting, he said, "There is one more thing that still has to be said."

"When you came out here and started working for us we discovered there was one attribute you had that we all learned from. Personal pride. You took the grounds here and turned them into a doggone country club. Everyone that visits here wants to know who is responsible, and we're very proud to tell them it's you."

"You did one other thing," he continued. "You did it for people that were not your friends, not your co-workers. But you did it for the inmates. Like usual, you jumped right in the middle, and to this day the outside inmate crew is thriving because of you, buddy."

Slowly Troy lifted his head and turned to look at everyone.

His lips formed a thank you, his eyes shone with gratitude. One at a time, people came over and stood or knelt beside his wheelchair to take their turn to speak to Troy. Many were aware that they were saying goodbye… knowing they would never see him again. Most of them wouldn't.

Once again, we experienced the pendulum of emotions as the day was filled with both great sadness and great joy. It was the balanced scales again.

§

By the time the middle of summer arrived, progress was still painfully slow on the house. Every month since May, the builder had promised "just one more month." We were at the end of our rope. I told the builder we were moving in, in August—no matter what. He was visibly a little shaken, but we noticed things started happening at an accelerated pace.

So on August 12th, my birthday, with the help once again of Troy's friends from Marion County, we moved in.

The house was not finished—the appliances weren't installed in the kitchen, the deck wasn't on (and that was a long drop to the ground!), and the den wasn't nearly finished, just to mention a few things. We spent the first several weeks in our new home as housemates of multiple sub-contractors. And, oh, the dust! But it was worth it. We were finally in our dream home. Together.

7
MINISTERING ANGELS

"Be not forgetful to entertain strangers:
for thereby some have entertained angels unawares."
(Hebrews 13:2 KJV)

White curtains surrounded us. Troy lay on the gurney, a white sheet draped over him. We were alone for the last few moments before they would take him into surgery.

"Just think of it as 'a walk in the park,'" I teased. I was trying hard to console him.

"Yeah," Troy said. "And I think I just stepped in something!" He could always come up with something better than I could for a good laugh.

Dr. Cohen was going to perform a cervical esophagostomy, a procedure where a permanent opening is made in the side of the neck, and a tube inserted. This was to become Troy's source of food for the remainder of his life. This was actually the second attempt to provide a feeding tube. The first surgery several months before had failed.

Moments before, the doctor had counseled us one last time. If Troy was ever going to have a tracheotomy done to go on a ventilator for life support, this would be the time to do it. A tracheotomy is another hole in the throat with tubing hooked up to a ventilator, a large machine that whirs and beeps and does your breathing for you. A tracheotomy requires regular suctioning as well as around the clock monitoring.

For most ALS victims, death comes when their lungs become too weak to function. Going on a ventilator to extend life is a huge decision, and is an option that only a small number of people with ALS choose. Ultimately, it means having a totally paralyzed body hooked up to life support. One of the problems is that it is still not a guarantee that life will continue. Because of the vulnerability of their systems, another common cause of death for ALS is pneumonia, which can happen even on a ventilator.

Stephen Hawking, world-renowned physicist, is one of the more famous ALS sufferers to have successfully extended his life on a ventilator.

Dr. Cohen knew that being under anesthesia in Troy's weakened condition was a significant risk. His breathing was already compromised. He would not likely survive a future surgery. If he was going to have the tracheotomy done, it was going to have to be now.

However, there was also the risk that if he had the tracheotomy done at this point, he may never be able to breathe on his own again. Because of the stress on his system from the surgery, he would need to go on the ventilator while he was recovering. And there was the chance that he wouldn't be able to get back off the life support.

We had already been over and over this issue. It's a huge decision. And a very personal one for each family to make. If it had been up to me, I would have done anything to keep Troy alive as long as possible. But in the end, it was his decision, and I had to keep quiet and respect that.

Troy had been firm that he did not want to be on a ventilator to keep him alive. We knew that Troy's lung capacity had already dropped to less than fifty percent of normal.

I was extremely relieved and thankful when he ultimately agreed to get the feeding tube. Without it, ALS sufferers are vulnerable to choking to death as well as starvation. The tongue and throat muscles weaken to the point where their swallowing can no longer be controlled. They can end up swallowing too soon and choke. Another problem is the food or liquids can go down the wrong channel and into the windpipe, causing problems in the lungs.

"It's better to get it sooner than later," Dr. Johnston, his neurologist had advised.

Good advice.

Troy agreed to the feeding tube—but that's where he drew the line.

§

The whole eating thing had become such a nightmare. First, because Troy's arm strength was one of the first things to go, he needed someone else to feed him. With his tongue and throat muscles weakening by the day, he had to chew everything carefully and laboriously. Meals became longer and longer to finish. Minimum two hours. It seemed like we would just finish one in time to start preparing for the next. His mom tried to make light of it.

"I never thought I'd be feeding you again!" she joked. "This is like old times."

Troy was not amused.

Eating was very tiring and discouraging for him. There was the constant fear of choking.

Choking had become commonplace, and we had learned not to panic. We both needed to stay calm as he worked to get control back.

I can remember one very warm summer evening before we moved into the house, when the temperature was still in the 90s. After several days of record-breaking heat (for Oregon!), we had to get out of that stifling apartment. We took one-year-old Victoria and went to the air-conditioned shopping mall. Apparently, a lot of other people had the same idea. It was a challenge just to find a table at the food court.

Thankfully, a couple, seeing Troy in the wheelchair with Victoria on his lap, gave us their table. I wheeled Troy up to the table and joined the long line at the counter. Every thirty seconds I was looking back to make sure he was ok. With Victoria under one arm, I juggled a tray of Caesar salads with the other.

By now, Troy was accustomed to being fed. We had grown used to the stares. The self-consciousness had given way to survival. It has given me a completely different perspective on people in wheelchairs.

It may have been the Caesar salad. Or maybe the extra tension and distraction of being in a public place. Eating for Troy took total concentration. At mealtimes we couldn't laugh, joke or even talk to him. He wanted no distractions. For a family that was used to sharing and laughing a lot at the dinner table, this was challenging. Especially with a one-year-old.

There were times when we would have to turn our head or hide behind our napkin to keep from laughing. We got into trouble more than once.

Whatever the reason this time, Troy started to choke on his food. Knowing the drill, I stood up and tried talking him through it.

The problem was that Victoria started choking too! Now what was I going to do?! I was mortified! Both of them choking?

Then it dawned on me what was happening—Victoria was copying her papa. She must have thought that since Troy was choking, she should too.

People started rushing over to help us. Embarrassed, I motioned them away, saying everyone was ok. Really. People looked at me like I was crazy, letting this poor child choke to death.

Once Troy gained his composure, we looked over at each other with a sigh of relief. Troy's face broke into a huge grin and I burst out laughing.

Another time it was pizza. It was Saturday and Mom was over at the apartment helping us. Troy had tried to order the pizza for us. But the guy on the other end of the phone couldn't understand him.

"Is this a joke?" he had asked and hung up the phone.

Troy was so frustrated and discouraged. It took all of my restraint not to go down to the pizza joint and strangle that kid with both hands!

Part way through dinner Troy choked on a bite of pizza. I tried to calm him down, but it was not working. He couldn't stop choking and everyone was starting to panic.

Mom called 911. Michelle, then eight years old, was told to take Victoria away from the horror. They went and locked themselves in the bathroom. I pulled him to his feet, and tried leaning him forward.

The paramedics poured into the apartment just as Troy managed to clear his airway. Thankfully, they were very nice and treated Troy with dignity. I could feel their sympathy as they realized what a tough situation we were in. One of them picked up Victoria and played with her for a minute so she would not be afraid of all these men storming our home.

At that point, Troy had to stop eating things that required chewing. His diet became one of pureed foods and liquids with a thickening agent added. Yogurt, cream of wheat, and tapioca pudding became daily staples. (I will never be able to make tapioca pudding again without thinking of Troy.)

Troy's muscles were atrophying down to next to nothing. He was dropping weight rapidly — by the time he went in to have the esophagostomy done, he weighed 138 pounds. In just a year and a half, he had lost 100 pounds. He looked like he had just come from a concentration camp.

The decision even to get a feeding tube was a tough decision. I struggled with the idea of the doctors putting a permanent hole in my husband's body. It was like it was some kind of disfigurement. There was no turning back once we did that. His body would never be the same again, and it brought yet another loss. However, in hindsight, we should have done it much sooner, before he actually needed it and was in such a weakened state.

Many ALS victims don't want to go through the surgery and its risks. For some, knowing they are going to die, a feeding tube only prolongs the inevitable. But for us, it meant that Troy wouldn't die prematurely from starvation. It was a practical decision as well, since it took the stress out of eating, making it so much easier on all of us.

Our pastor, Ron Mehl, came to our home to help us with this decision. He shared with us that he, too, had a "permanent hole" near his collarbone where the doctors administered chemotherapy for his leukemia.

Hearing about this somehow gave Troy and me the courage to go ahead with the surgery.

That had been in May of 1995, while we were still living in the apartment, one year after his diagnosis. At that point we scheduled the first surgery at OHSU. The normal procedure for a feeding tube for ALS patients is called a gastro intestinal or GI tube. It is an outpatient surgery where a short tube is inserted directly into the stomach.

Troy hated hospitals. He was one of those guys who grew weak in the knees just drawing blood for a routine blood test. The prospect of being back in the hospital, even for just a day, was enough to make him turn and run.

Only he couldn't. I was in control of the wheelchair! And he was stuck.

Because he was unable to communicate with anyone but me, the doctors made an exception, and let me come into the operating room. I put on one of those blue doctor gowns and surgical caps. In his usual way, Troy was making everyone laugh with his jokes. Of course, I would hear the joke before anyone else since I was doing the translating because of his slurred speech. I refused to finish translating one of his remarks when I realized he was making fun of the way I looked!

Dr. Fennerly arrived and explained everything to us. The anesthetic was put into his IV. Within moments Troy was out. It was time for me to go... and wait.

I went to sit in the waiting room, absent-mindedly leafing through a worn magazine. Within fifteen minutes the doctor walked into the room. I was surprised to see him so soon. Had an hour gone by that fast? Dr. Fennerly was tall and good-looking like Troy, and around the same age. He walked over to me, and asked me to come out in the hall. I can still remember his exact words.

"I'm so sorry. I cannot believe this happened! It only happens once in a blue moon..."

"What? What? Just tell me," I thought to myself.

"We were not able to put in the tube," the doctor said. He explained that once in "a blue moon" they run into this situation where the stomach is positioned in such a way that they are unable to put the tube in.

"I'm so sorry," he said again. "He should be able to go home in a couple hours after the anesthetic wears off."

I could not believe what I was hearing.

No feeding tube? What were we going to do?! The thought of watching Troy starve to death was more than I could bear. Sitting alone in the waiting room, powerless to stop the tears streaming down my face, I cried out to God.

"Lord, what now? We have been through so much. Why this? What about the part that you will never leave us or forsake us?" My anguish turned into anger and then to fear.

"Marilyn, Dr. Fennerly called and told me what happened. I came right down." I looked up to see Dr. Johnston, our neurologist, heading over to me. She sat down next to me and handed over a tissue. She explained in more detail what had gone wrong with the surgery.

"However, there is an alternative. It isn't used very often, and we haven't done it with an ALS patient. But there is another place a feeding tube can be put in," she said.

She went on to explain about a procedure called an esophagostomy. An opening is made in the side of the neck (a permanent hole!), and a long tube is inserted that goes directly to the stomach.

My tears started all over again as fresh hope welled up inside. I knew that God had been with me all along, and had just answered my prayer. And at that moment, Dr. Johnston looked just like an angel.

Troy was taken to a room in another part of the hospital while he recovered from the failed surgery. When Troy woke up another surgeon came to see us and explain more about the esophagostomy. Troy agreed to the surgery, and the doctor was able to arrange to do it the next day at noon.

The doctor recommended that Troy stay the night in the hospital. Like I said, he hated hospitals, and he didn't want to stay a minute more than he had to.

"We're going home," he told me. "We can come back in the morning."

The next morning I packed some things into a suitcase. This time it was going to be a two to three night stay in the hospital — for both of us. Troy wanted me with him every minute. I couldn't even leave to get a cup of coffee. Not that the coffee in a hospital is worth drinking, but anything would have helped with the little to no sleep I was existing on. But I didn't want to leave him.

I would stay at his side twenty-four hours a day. No one else could communicate with him. It was a terrifying thing for him to be in a hospital with tubes and monitors, and not be able to ask for help. A call monitor was set up that he could operate with his foot since he had no use of his arms or hands. But even when the nurse came he couldn't tell them what he needed. His pillow would need adjusting so that he didn't feel like he couldn't breath. Or his saliva needed suctioning. Or any one of a hundred other things that had become routine for me.

Victoria had spent the night with the Williams, a dear family that took care of her during the days I was at work. Paula Williams was such a source of strength and comfort to me during these days. I remember the first time I saw Paula after we got the diagnosis. I drove over to her house to drop off little Victoria, and she met me at the car. Standing there on the sidewalk, not saying a word, she put her arms around me and we cried together.

It was just what I needed. Not someone telling me everything was going to be okay. Not someone telling me that I was going to have to be strong. But a friend who felt my pain and shared it with me.

Paula knew what we were facing more than I did. She had helped take care of a man with ALS from her church. She had watched his two-year deterioration and death. This was not just a death sentence. It was a hideous prison sentence as well.

For the trip back to the hospital the next morning, Troy wanted to take his sports car since it was just the two of us. It was a chilly spring morning as I put his coat on him, and ran out to the car. I threw the suitcase in the trunk, and pulled the car up to the curb. The sidewalk was wet with rain that had now slowed to a soft mist. A heavy cloud cover hid the sun from showing its face. I ran back to get Troy.

At this point he could still walk, very slowly, with someone helping him. His leg muscles lasted longer than most of his other muscles. Taking hold of his arm, I held him steady with one hand and locked the apartment door with the other. We made our way slowly down the sidewalk, Troy's arms hanging limp at his side. I would hold onto one of his arms with both hands. His upper body bent slightly forward, he would shuffle along, unable to lift his feet very far off the ground. Getting in and out of the sports car was quite a production, but I wanted to give Troy any small amount of satisfaction I could.

As usual, Troy was quiet on the way to the hospital. I knew he was dreading this. His eyes portrayed the battle he was having with his fear and apprehension.

We pulled into the all too familiar parking garage. *Yes!* I thought to myself. *A parking space not far from the elevators.* Getting out of the car, I went around to Troy's side. Getting him out was not a whole lot easier than getting him in, but we had our routine worked out. I lifted one leg out, then the other. Crossing his arms on his lap, I made sure his head was tilted forward so it would not drop back. There were times when I would forget that part. With weak neck muscles, he couldn't stop his head from falling backwards. Poor guy! His head would just dangle backwards like a rag doll until I could rescue him.

Taking hold of both arms just underneath the armpits, I would rock him forward. The first lift was to get him swung around to face out the door. Then I would put one of my feet between his for balance and the other one back for leverage. On the count of three, using a rocking motion, I would lift him to his feet. I walked him the few steps to the back of the car to wait while I got the suitcase out of the trunk. Setting the suitcase on the concrete floor, I went around to my side of the car to lock the door.

I don't know if he was getting anxious or just trying to help me out, but Troy started to take a few steps on his own towards the elevator.

My back was turned and I didn't see what was going on. But I heard it… the most sickening sound I have ever heard. Troy lost his balance and fell straight back, helpless to stop himself or cushion the fall. His head was the first thing to hit the concrete.

"No!!!!," I screamed as I dropped to my knees beside him. Blood was rapidly pooling around his head.

"God, please…please don't let him die! Not here. Not like this," I prayed.

"Somebody help us!" I screamed into the empty parking garage.

A woman suddenly appeared out of nowhere. Calmly she knelt down beside me. She asked me what happened as she stripped off her jacket.

"He…he fell," I stuttered, sobbing hysterically. "He can't talk and he can't move!" I managed to say.

There was a time when I would be the calm one in a crisis. But not anymore. There had been too many of them, too much adrenaline used up. She took her jacket, and putting it under his head, she cradled his head in her hands to try to stop the bleeding.

Just then, two security guys in brown uniforms showed up in their security cart. One of them grabbed his radio and called 911 while the other wheeled the cart around to go stop traffic.

Troy calmed down as this kind woman held his head and reassured him.

I paced.

Where are they?! What is taking so long? The security guard called again.

"They're on their way, Ma'am," he said. "Emergency is right across the street."

He didn't know what was taking so long either. He left to go see if he could see them coming for us. It took twenty minutes before the guards yelled down, "They're here!"

The ambulance screeched to a halt. Out piled six to eight men and women. They circled around us as the woman with the clipboard knelt down and started asking questions.

"Can't we just get him to the hospital and ask questions on the way?" I pleaded.

"No, this is procedure," she callously replied.

Barely able to contain myself I answered her questions about date of birth, insurance, allergies, medical condition, etc., etc. They finally loaded Troy into the ambulance and I climbed in beside him. We literally drove less than half a block! Basically, out of the parking garage and across the street. I could have carried him there faster!

Remembering the woman who had helped us, I turned to find her to thank her. She was gone. The last time I saw her was when the ambulance arrived. She had stood up and I remember seeing blood all over her sweater and her hands. Still today, I can't help but wonder if maybe she was actually an angel, one of several sent to help us.

When we got there, one of the paramedics pulled me aside and apologized for his co-worker's rudeness. "That was uncalled for," he said. "You have enough to deal with." Other than on this one occasion, I had found the ambulance crews and paramedics to be nothing short of fantastic.

His mom arrived almost faster than the ambulance and met us in emergency. We stood together, arms around each other, and watched as they did a CT scan. Miraculously there was only a slight concussion and head wound. I held his hand as they put in several stitches.

"Sorry, Hon," he said weakly, managing a smile.

Behind the curtain in the bed next to us, a doctor was just finishing up. Walking around the curtain, he spotted us and his mouth dropped open.

"What on earth are you doing here?!" Dr. Fennerly asked. It was the same doctor who, less than twenty-four hours before, had done the surgery for the GI tube. "Boy, do you have bad luck!" he exclaimed.

Troy wanted to say something. The doctor waited patiently as I leaned over to hear what Troy was trying to say:

"At least…

it was not…

my nose…

this time," Troy joked. With all we went through, Troy never lost his sense of humor or that wonderful smile.

Five months went by before Troy agreed to go back to the hospital again for the feeding tube surgery…

§

"Okay, we're ready for him," said the nurse, gently pulling back the white curtain. I walked alongside him as two orderlies and the nurse wheeled Troy down a long hallway toward the double doors. Dr. Cohen met us at the doors.

"Are you ready, big guy?" he asked. Troy looked towards me. He wanted to say something.

"Can my wife come?" I interpreted for him.

"Not this time, I'm afraid," said the doctor.

I kissed him on the cheek, and managed a smile, holding back the tears as hard as I could. His eyes locked onto mine as the doors swung open and they wheeled him through. As the doors closed behind them, I stood there alone, and let the tears flow once again.

8
SIX MONTHS AND COUNTING...

"God calls the unqualified to do the impossible."
~Author unknown

"I'm not ready to go yet!"

It was supposed to be a three-day stay in the hospital. But Troy wanted out. So we ended up going home after one night. From the moment he started to wake up from the surgery until he got home, it was absolute torture for him.

I had spent the long hours of the operation in a small waiting room reserved for the families of surgery patients. At first, there was only one other person there as I sat and prayed, and tried to pass the time. After an hour or so, a small, elderly gentleman walked in. He was wearing a worn, brown tweed suit and cap, with small wire rimmed glasses perched on his nose. He was carrying a brief case, one that had certainly seen better days. He proceeded to set the briefcase down, and open it.

He smiled at me and started chattering away. Oddly, I cannot remember what it was he was talking about. Or even what was in the briefcase. It had nothing to do with waiting for someone to come out of surgery. But he continued a lively conversation, smiling the whole time, as if he didn't have a care in the world. He looked like the angel, Clarence, in the movie "It's a Wonderful Life," one of Troy's all-time favorites.

Our conversation helped the time pass quickly, and before I knew it, the hospital phone on the wall rang with the news that Troy was out of surgery. "Clarence" politely stood up, shut his briefcase, and tipped his hat to me. With that, he left.

When I arrived in the recovery room, Troy was a wreck. Two nurses were working on him, checking vital signs, etc. In his eyes was total panic. He was trying desperately to communicate something to me. I could tell by looking at him that because of his panicking he was choking and couldn't breathe.

I tried desperately to get the nurses to help him, but they said that he was okay, he wasn't really choking. Because he was still heavily medicated, he would then go back into an unconscious state. The moment he would wake up, the panic would set in again.

His mom came to the hospital when she got off work. She had trouble locating us (no surprise at that hospital!). When she finally found out where we were, she was told she could not go in there. She went in anyway. She arrived just as he was being wheeled out of recovery to go to his room. One look at him was more than she could bear. It was the worst she had ever seen him.

The nurses and I wheeled him into his room. It was a huge ordeal trying to transfer him to the bed. He was thrashing and flailing, but it was on the inside, because he couldn't move his body. He was desperate to breathe. Mom had to leave the room.

"He was so distraught!" she recalls. As she stood out in the hall, leaning against the wall, she felt so helpless. "I wanted to hit somebody, to tell them to make him feel better!"

It was a long, sleepless night.

At Troy's insistence, we went home the next day. It was against the better judgment of the doctors. Later that night, I would wonder, too, if we hadn't made a huge mistake. I was in way over my head, trying to figure out how to use this new tube (even though they had given me a crash course at the hospital), care for the wound in his neck from the surgery, deal with his extreme discomfort, nausea…you name it! If it hadn't been for Lucy, I probably would have loaded him into the car and gone back to the hospital.

Lucy and Mike Sawyer had become such amazing and faithful friends. Lucy had offered to come over when we got back from the hospital. I called and took her up on her offer, and she arrived that afternoon.

There we were in the kitchen, Troy in his wheelchair with his laptop computer next to him on a TV tray. What a team Lucy and I made! Actually, we were more like Laurel and Hardy.

Poor Troy! He was trying to communicate something to me. He finally spelled out on his computer, "Lucy is burning something in the microwave!"

She and I were so busy trying to read the instructions on all this feeding tube paraphernalia that we hadn't noticed the smoke.

Lucy had put our dinner in the microwave and set it for thirty minutes instead of three! We had a good laugh over that one.

Next was our trial run at Troy's first "meal." It was a can of Jevity, a liquid food that we were to put through a syringe into his tube. I had been carefully reading the instructions, and unwrapping all the supplies that were wrapped in sterile plastic. It was very intimidating to put something into a tube that you knew was going directly into his stomach. Or at least I hoped that's where it would end up!

I took a deep breath, and said, "Okay, here it goes."

I pushed on the syringe and nothing happened. I tried pushing a little harder. Still nothing. By then, Troy was trying to say something.

Getting flustered, I told him to hold on, I could do this.

Troy was getting more anxious to tell me something. I stopped and waited as he worked to get his words formed.

"Take the cap off the syringe," he said with a grin on his face. Lucy and I laughed until we cried.

§

By now it was mid-September, one month after moving into our glorious new home. The newness hadn't worn off even the slightest bit. We were still on our honeymoon.

Every morning when I woke up to that breathtaking, expansive view, it felt like being on top of the world. Troy loved the front row seat we had to the sky and all its weather patterns. The clouds were a continual show on a windy day.

Oh, and the lights at night! That was an added bonus we hadn't even known about until our first night in the house. Up until then, we had only seen the property in the daylight. At night, there is a completely new landscape of city lights.

Another surprise awaited us that first night in the house. We had been asleep for a few hours when I was awakened by the sound of a car coming up the gravel drive. Troy had heard it too. I looked at the clock and saw that it was past midnight.

The car was moving slowly. We heard it come to a stop in front of the house. My heart started to pound. I knew that I would have to investigate. It was excruciating for Troy, who by nature was a protector, to have his wife have to be the one to confront the unknown.

I crept out of bed without turning on any lights. Our bedroom was right off the foyer by the front entrance, which was a set of double doors with glass framed in each door. I could see from the bedroom doorway a flashlight shining in through the glass doors. I knew that if I turned on a light I would be in full view as soon as I stepped out of the bedroom door. Instead, I crept along the wall towards the door, trying to avoid the flashlight.

As soon as I got close to the front door, I saw the red lights on top of the car parked out front. It was a police officer! I switched on the outside light and opened the door.

"I was just checking to make sure everything was alright," he said. "We got a call from 911, and when we called back no one answered. That's when we go and investigate."

"But we didn't call 911," I said.

He double-checked our phone number, and sure enough, that was ours. Then it dawned on me! Our "medic alert" phone was programmed to dial 911 if it was activated. Apparently there was a short in the new wiring that set off the phone. We didn't have a phone set up in the bedroom yet, so we hadn't heard when the 911 operator had tried to call back.

It would happen twice more before we got it fixed properly. The Newberg police department got to know who we were in a short amount of time. Thankfully, they were very understanding. And it was not very long before the Newberg hospital emergency and the fire department would get to know us as well.

Our first trip to the Newberg hospital emergency was when Troy's feeding tube got clogged. A lot of the medicine had to be crushed and mixed in water in order to go through the tube, not to mention a ton of different vitamins he was taking.

When we arrived, the doctor on duty had never done this procedure before. Not surprising — it's not your ordinary emergency case! Fortunately, they did have the right size feeding tube in stock. So between the doctor, the nurse, and myself we figured out what to do. After that, I kept a supply of them at home and did it myself.

§

With only two months before winter would set in, Troy got busy on the landscaping. He spent a good part of his day at his computer working on the landscape drawings, plant lists, and instructions for me. He kept assuring me that it would be a "low maintenance" plan. Yeah, right!

Even I could tell that wasn't the case when I saw the size of the lawn he wanted to put in. He affectionately came up with a new nickname for me—he told everyone his "Deere" wife had turned into the "Lawn Ranger." Go ahead—groan. We usually did at most of his jokes.

Then there was the huge rose garden. Not to mention the shrubs, and the perennials, and the ornamental grasses, and the flowering trees, and the hedges, and the bank of groundcover roses. But I have to admit it was stunning. He had a remarkable sense of design.

At first, he was able to go along on the trips to the nurseries to pick out the plants. And man, he was picky! Inevitably, the shrub or tree he would want would be way down the row. I would drag it over to his wheelchair for inspection, and then drag it back again when it wasn't quite right.

Troy would supervise the placement and the planting to make sure it was done right. Lots of people volunteered to help. We had several days when we had a whole crew of helpers sprawled out across our property.

One time it was my whole office staff, another was a local church, and then a youth group from another church. The landscaping was rapidly taking shape. That became the next goal. To get the landscaping in while Troy was still here to see his dream realized.

Troy liked to use boulders in landscaping, which usually required equipment to move them. One day we had a track-hoe, an expensive piece of heavy equipment, to place several large boulders. Wearing sunglasses and sitting in his wheelchair in the driveway, Troy directed the two workers on how he wanted the boulders positioned.

The clock was running at $120 an hour. But it was important that Troy had the final say in how it should look. I stood next to Troy and asked the questions while the workers waited for his reactions.

I had learned we could communicate a lot faster by asking "yes and no" questions.

Eyebrows up meant "yes," eyebrows down "no."

"Troy, is that okay?" Eyebrows down.

"So which one isn't right? The middle one?" Eyebrows down.

"The one on the left?" Eyebrows down.

"The one on the right?" Still down.

"Do you want it turned?" Eyebrows up.

"Do you want it turned to the left?" Eyebrows down.

"Okay, do you want it turned to the right?" Eyebrows down.

"Well, there are not a lot of options left, Troy." My patience was running a little short by now.

One of the workers yelled, "Maybe he wants them all switched around."

"Okay, so do you want the whole thing moved further toward the road, Troy?" Eyebrows up, several times, enthusiastically.

The workers and I broke out in applause and laughter.

§

The wheelchair that had become Troy's new way of getting around was a power chair that, at first, he could operate himself. We had it equipped with a joystick control. Even though he had very little function left in his arms and hands, he had just enough to operate the sensitive black ball that steered the chair. His arm would rest on the armrest and I would put his cupped hand on top of the ball. He would give little Victoria rides around the house. I put her on his lap, put his free arm around her, and off they would go.

He managed to get around pretty well, at least for the first month or two. Except for the time he got stuck in the deep gravel at the big curve in the driveway. I had to drive down with our handicap-equipped van to get him. There was no way I could push him up the hill manually. That chair was heavy! Sometimes his hand would get stuck on the joy stick, making the chair go around in circles. The first time it happened I thought he was just playing around, "cutting cookies" in the gravel. But one look at his face told me he wasn't doing it for fun.

§

We now had to have help for Troy when I was away at work. It started out on a part-time basis while we were still in the apartment. Our first caregiver came for a couple of hours a day on the days that Summer, Mike, or I weren't there. Mainly we needed someone to feed him and give him his medications.

The increasing need for caregivers was one of our greatest challenges. Finding the right people, training them, and then keeping them was an on-going problem in the beginning. We started out using an agency. The first young woman they sent us worked out well. Troy and I liked her, and we were relieved that maybe this wasn't going to be as bad as we thought. But then one day, all of a sudden, they sent someone else. We didn't find out until later that our first caregiver had a relative involved in the Oklahoma City bombing, and had left to go back to Oklahoma.

The next several they sent were not so great, and we didn't always know who was going to show up. The agency had to use a couple different people to cover the schedule.

Eventually they found a woman who was able to commit to the days we needed, and she was a joy. Her name was Marvina, and she wasn't afraid to take Troy out to places he wanted to go. Michelle remembers going to movies with her dad and Marvina during that summer in the apartment, and how much fun it was to do "normal things." But Marvina told us that she was going back to nursing school in the fall, and wouldn't be able to keep working for us.

We felt like we were back at square one. We would have to go through the search all over again, not to mention the training involved. By the time Marvina left, we had just moved into the new house. We needed someone who could handle the feeding tube and the difficult job of communicating with Troy. So many of the caregivers didn't have the patience to let him say what it was he wanted — and how he wanted it.

Troy had told me early on in the illness that one of his biggest fears was being invisible, treated by people as if he wasn't there. The thought of being with people, but not being included in the conversation was really tough for him. I always made a point of including him even though at times it was very slow, and required a great deal of patience.

After Marvina was Rachel. Of course, Marvina was a hard act to follow. Rachel was only twenty years old, had strawberry blonde hair, and was very sweet (most of the time). The thing I will always remember about Rachel, though, were her driving skills…

Friday mornings were the day we took the garbage can down to the bottom of the long driveway. I was getting ready to go to work, and asked Rachel if she would mind taking the suburban and driving the garbage down. A few minutes later, she came rushing through the kitchen door, out of breath.

"There's something you've got to see," she stammered. "It's the car. I got it stuck in the side of the house!"

"Wait, wait, hold on," I said. "You did what?"

"Just come outside," she pleaded, now in tears.

She ran back outside with me close behind. Sure enough. I hadn't heard wrong. The suburban was stuck in the side of the house! The engine was still running.

"Rachel, how on earth did you do this?" I asked in disbelief. I stood there looking in amazement at our suburban. The running board on the passenger side was wedged deep into the siding across the corner of the house. The stucco was crumbled and the wood 2x4s beneath the stucco were splintered. The passenger door was caved in.

"I don't know how I did it!" she tearfully replied. "I guess I cut the corner too close when I was trying to back up, and then when I hit the house, I tried pulling forward. I think that's when the running board got stuck."

I climbed in and turned the engine off. After a closer inspection, I decided I had better call a tow truck and not risk further damage. You should have seen the look on the tow truck driver's face!

"How are we going to tell Troy?" Rachel said. She was now sobbing uncontrollably

"Rachel, honey, don't worry about it. It will be okay," I said, trying to console her. I, too, was wondering how Troy was going to react.

"Why don't I go tell him, and you just sit here in the kitchen, and try to get a hold of yourself."

When I went in and told Troy the story of what had happened, I was relieved and thankful for his reaction. Instead of getting upset, he smiled in amusement.

"It's just a car," he spelled out on his computer.

You know, really, what's a car, or a little corner of the house, after what we had been through? Our priorities had changed dramatically as a result of living with a terminal illness.

§

Between teenage drivers and nurses, we had a whole trunk full of car stories. I'm not sure which one was more memorable, Rachel and the suburban or Flo and the old Pontiac.

Flo was a hospice volunteer who came every Wednesday morning for a couple of hours to help out. Even though we had discovered that we were the same age, Flo had just gotten her driver's license a few months before. After all these years, she decided she needed to be able to drive occasionally. I don't think she ever ventured outside of Newberg. She just stayed on the familiar streets.

We had just put down some extra gravel on the big curve in the driveway. Because it was somewhat steep, some cars tended to spin their tires and kick the gravel off to the side.

The next day when Flo arrived for her usual Wednesday morning routine, she got her car stuck in the deep gravel as she was starting around the curve. I could hear her tires spinning in the gravel from inside the house. I watched out the bedroom window as she started backing the car down the driveway. Normally, that would have been the right thing to do. But backing up can be tricky for inexperienced drivers.

I watched in dismay as she turned the wheels the wrong way and was headed for the embankment. I raced out to the deck to yell down at her to stop just in time to see the back wheels of her car go over the bank. She stopped the car with the front tires still barely clinging to the driveway. As she opened her door and stood up, I yelled down to her to make sure the emergency brake was on. Just then the car broke loose and rolled backwards. Flo had been standing next to the open door, and as the car started to roll, the door knocked her flat on her back, and rolled over her. I watched in horror as the whole scene unfolded, as if in slow motion. The car came to a stop about a hundred feet down the slope.

"Flo!" I screamed. "Don't move. I'm coming!"

My legs flew down the hill. I found her sitting up, dazed. The front tire had run over her head. There was literally a tire track across her face. Her glasses were smashed, and her forehead cut. Remarkably her broken glasses hadn't done any damage to her face.

I put my arm around her shoulders and we prayed and cried. She wanted to get to the house and call her supervisor so I helped her up, and walked her slowly up the driveway. (I learned later that was not the right thing to do. I never should have let her move.)

Her supervisor arrived and took her straight to the hospital. Miraculously, there was nothing broken. Except for two black eyes, and some cuts, she would be fine. The miraculous stories of God's protection kept growing.

§

Our follow-up visit to Dr. Cohen a month after the feeding tube surgery was encouraging. Even though Troy hadn't started to gain any weight back yet, the weight loss had been stopped and we finally had him up to enough calories a day that he could at least maintain his weight.

The best news was that he had gained strength back.

And the problem of excess saliva had decreased. We had a portable suction machine that we used regularly to help him manage the saliva since he couldn't swallow.

It was one of the few times during the relentless progression of the disease that something had actually improved. Dr. Cohen told Dr. Johnston that he was very pleased with how well Troy was doing since the surgery.

Our tiny ray of hope got a little brighter.

But the roller coaster continued. By December, two months later, he had started going downhill again. His neck muscles were getting weaker and weaker. He could no longer lift his head, and would sit in his wheelchair with his head hanging over his lap. It was tiring for him, and difficult to communicate. When he had visitors, he couldn't look at them unless I held his head for him. We tried all kinds of methods of propping his head up for him.

Marvina's husband, Ross, even welded together a pulley of sorts that attached to the back of his wheelchair. We made a headband sling for his forehead to rest in, and then using the pulley we could raise or lower his head.

But still, nothing worked. All these different neck braces and systems made him feel like he was choking. The only way for his throat to stay open was to lean his head forward, or if he was lying in bed with his head to one side. During the night he required suctioning regularly. Neither of us was getting enough sleep and we were exhausted.

Still, we had resolved to make the most of whatever time we had left. We didn't know how much time that was. We were now past the predicted time from both Dr. Johnston and Dr. Edwards. We still hung on to the hope that maybe Troy would hold on long enough for a cure to be found. Or maybe God would do a miracle and heal him.

Whatever the outcome, whatever the timing, our goal was still to be victorious. Our victory was not whether Troy lived or died from ALS. Our victory would be in never giving up hope, in preserving and strengthening our marriage through this adversity, and in living every day as best we could, however many or few they were. Our victory was never losing our faith.

§

It was December 24th, Christmas Eve. Everyone else in the house was asleep. Troy's legs started to stiffen, and his breathing was becoming increasingly labored. The harder it was to breathe, the more he panicked. I feared he would not make it through the night.

But somehow he made it through to Christmas morning, and was finally able to relax enough to get some sleep. I called the doctor. Convinced that Troy would die within weeks, or days, Dr. Johnston referred us to hospice, a team of professionals who specialize in end of life comfort care rather than a cure. In order to qualify for hospice, a doctor needs to indicate that a patient has less than six months to live.

The nurse arrived the next day. I had feared it would be just one more resource, one more professional that I would have to go through all the history and red tape with. Instead, hospice was just what we needed.

For the first time, I had a team that could orchestrate all our needs. They became our central resource instead of having to go through several people to accomplish all our different needs, such as equipment, medications, nursing care, etc. If I had to call someone in the middle of the night, they were there. I didn't have to go through a doctor's answering service. We put them on speed dial on every phone in the house.

It was through hospice that Troy was first prescribed morphine. It was what he needed to calm the panic that would set in when his breathing became difficult, and it eased some of the pain in his neck and shoulders.

The day after Christmas, after the nurse left, Troy typed on his computer:

"I'm not ready to go yet. I don't want to leave you. I love you. I feel so cheated that we barely got started. So many dreams, so many experiences yet undone. So many things we have not shared. That is the hardest thing."

And then he added, "Always remember all I want is to do God's will and to have his will done."

9
WALKING THROUGH IT

*"Even though I walk through the valley of the shadow of death,
I fear no evil, for You are with me…"*
(Psalm 23:4 NASB)

Where does the living stop and the dying begin?

"Marilyn, you've got to accept the fact that Troy is dying," Dr. Johnston would tell me.

"Well, have you?" I snapped back. "Have you accepted the fact that you're dying?"

We are all dying—or we are living. The end result is the same for everyone. What we do with the space in-between birth and death determines the legacy we leave. Troy's legacy was a life lived to its fullest, to its last breath.

Anyone given a terminal diagnosis is faced with the question: How are you supposed to prepare to die? Do you try to do all the things you have always wanted to do, but put off? Do you spend money like crazy and get it all as fast as you can?

Usually you are given a date, an educated guess, or a statistically charted prognosis. But it's a moving target. It might speed up, and then slow down. You end up feeling as if you are going in circles. But the clock never stops ticking.

Maybe instead of getting all those things you always wanted, you stop spending. What's the point in buying that stuff anyway? You won't need those things before long. It would be a waste of money, right?

Do you stop exercising, eating right, or caring about what toxic chemicals you may be putting into your body? Does it matter? Your body isn't going to be around very long anyway.

Or do you exercise like Arnold Schwarzeneger, trying to outrun the illness? There is every kind of imaginable treatment option out there, and I think we tried half of them! When you are given a diagnosis of a disease where there is no known cause or cure, you start looking for one.

Every day we were faced with little decisions and big ones, based on this question. Do we live our lives as dying or living?

We tried both ways. Within a month of receiving the death sentence, Troy went out and bought the red convertible sports car. Now, I've seen guys in their mid forties do this, but Troy was only 32. His life was now on fast forward.

Our life became a whirlwind of naturopaths, nutritionists, herbalists, acupuncture specialists, chiropractors, physical therapists, speech therapists, occupational therapists, and an entourage of traditional medical doctors.

Needless to say, precious little time was left each day for living.

I remember a dear friend of mine, Joyce giving me the advice that we should live each day to its fullest, and to appreciate each day we had together. I just wasn't sure how to live each day to its fullest. In time, I would learn what profound advice this was. And another thing Joyce said…

"As hard as this is, your relationship with Troy will grow to a level few ever experience." She was right about that, too.

"Pull the shades down on the sun,
Don't wanna see the morning break into
another day I don't have the strength to face.

Close the door and keep it shut;
Lord, this ache is just too much for me to take.
How do I begin to pray my way back
To some kind of peace of mind?..."

It is hard to say when exactly it happened, but a shift took place in our attitude. There was no defining moment, but I observed it in both of us. We decided that no matter what happened or what anyone told us, we would keep living...keep growing...keep loving.

And there is a truth which I learned through all of this that is etched in me forever: that we never, ever, can know what the future will bring.

"...But then I hear love whispering through
The darkest of times
'You'll get through this
You'll break new ground
When you're lost within your weakness
Hope is waiting to be found.

You'll get through this
No matter what it takes
I believe in you for heaven's sake,
You'll get through this,'"[1]

No more hesitation on whether to buy a piece of equipment that he may only use a month or two. No more putting plans on hold for a birthday party or a graduation

---

[1] Words from the song "You'll Get Through This" by Ty Lacy

celebration, wondering if Troy would still be with us. (Troy was with us for three of our daughters' graduations, from kindergarten to college!). No more second-guessing how much time we had left. None of the doctors had been right anyway. It was really a huge relief when we came to this conclusion. It felt so much better to focus on living! Living comes so much more naturally than dying.

We were not very good at the dying part anyway, even though we tried to do the practical things such as drawing up a will and choosing a cemetery.

Now there was an interesting experience! If you are married, you will appreciate this. Here we are, driving around this huge cemetery in our specially equipped handicap van, pouring down rain. The cemetery, located in the hills of Portland, is a picturesque cemetery, one of the city's largest. Tall, old growth fir trees tower overhead. Mossy, concrete headstones tell the stories of those who have gone years before.

We drove around with the "plot salesperson" in the back of our van, a huge map spread across the seat. The windshield wipers were going full speed as she directed us up this hill and down that one, all the while pointing out the "features and benefits" (Hey, I used to sell real estate, so I can understand).

There was a historic area with more ornate tombstones, or perhaps we would prefer a quiet, shady knoll? And we're supposed to agree on where we want our final move to be?!

Two more trips, one dragging the family along after church, and we finally picked a spot. Of course, Troy could not actually go in his wheelchair and inspect all these potential spots. I would hike up the hill, carefully stepping around the grave markers. (Is it okay to actually step on a grave, or are there some kind of rules here?) When I would get to the spot, map in hand, I would wave my arms and point.

Once that was finally settled, the next step was the head stone. Troy had already designed one on his computer. It was to be a large cross, made of black marble.

One of his favorite Bible verses was to be inscribed on the front: "Above all else, guard your heart, for it is the wellspring of life" (Proverbs 4:23).

Sitting in our den, our "plot lady" (who, by the way, was very nice) was filling out paperwork and asking questions.

Troy would slowly type out his answer on the computer, using his foot to operate the mouse. Then the computer "voice" would say his answers.

She asked Troy how he would like his middle name, initials or full name.

He typed out "N.A."

His middle name is Norris, so I thought maybe he hit the "A" key by mistake.

He grinned and insisted it should be N.A.

"Maybe he is trying to say 'not applicable,'" she offered.

Seeing the twinkle in his eye, I asked, "What's the 'A' for, Hon?"

He typed out the letters, and the computer voice said "Awesome."

We broke out laughing. Troy could make us laugh even in the most "delicate" situations.

In the end, I found a little pioneer cemetery just a mile from our house with a view of four mountains. It was perfect. We cancelled the contract on the Portland cemetery.

When you think about it, is death itself a choice? No, it is the same for all of us.

However, choosing the time of our death is an option in some people's minds. But choosing the time of our death is no more natural to humanity than choosing the time of our birth.

It is a decision that is too big for us mortals. We don't have the perspective of the future that our Creator has.

As Troy would say, "He is the author and finisher of our lives."

That quote would come to be heard around the world.

10
JOSH

"Friendship is one mind in two bodies."
~Mencius

Josh came into our lives like a fresh, warm wind. Invigorating, strong, energetic, and full of fun. I could not have guessed it, but Josh was just what we needed.

Josh showed up at the door for his interview in the spring of 1996. It was March 14th to be exact, the day of our fourth wedding anniversary. It was hard to imagine that it had been only four years ago that Troy and I had been at the altar together. We had lived and experienced so much as husband and wife in these few years. It was like our marriage was on fast forward, as if we were now in our "golden years." My husband was now "retired" and at home where we could spend more time together, health declining as the end of his life neared. Only he was not 75... he was only 34 years old.

We had been desperately searching for another caregiver after Rachel quit in February. The agency was at a loss to find someone to do the number of hours we now needed, at the level of care that was required.

Since Troy had gone on morphine in addition to the feeding tube, the agency could no longer send someone with just a CNA license. It now needed to be a more skilled nurse, and with that the cost doubled.

In working with our insurance company, the case manager agreed to let us hire privately and pay their salary using the benefit that was normally for a skilled nursing facility. It was a huge relief, and it was a big savings for the insurance company, as well as us. This way we didn't have to use a registered nurse as required by an agency. It gave us much greater flexibility and control.

The challenge was finding someone. We had heard horror stories about putting ads in the paper. Instead, we sought help from people we knew to locate someone.

After being off work for three weeks with no one but me who was capable of taking care of Troy, I was getting discouraged and scared. The few leads we had received hadn't panned out. I knew that Troy was feeling like a huge burden. He felt responsible for my exhausted state, and yet helpless to do anything.

When I opened the front door that morning and first met Josh, I had no idea what an amazing relationship would develop between this young man and our family.

Here he was, only twenty-three years old. He was dressed in jeans, a flannel shirt, and hiking boots. Oh, and an earring. I was used to nurses and caregivers showing up in some kind of white uniform with a nametag.

Not Josh.

When I brought Josh into the den to meet Troy, he seemed so relaxed. His face didn't portray the shock and discomfort so many did at the first sight of Troy. Josh listened calmly as I explained the situation.

He shared with me later that he was "blown away" by my frankness in stating the obvious (that, and Troy's "amazing" entertainment center!). We told him Troy had an unknown amount of time left to live. That it could be as long as three months or a matter of a few weeks.

Josh had to make a decision about leaving a secure job at a nursing home for an unknown future with us. We were elated when he called back a few days later with his decision to come to work for us.

Josh brought not only his nursing skills, but also his fun loving spirit and positive attitude. And he brought another masculine presence into a household that was overwhelmingly female! I loved this young man from the moment I met him.

Troy finally had a caregiver and companion who shared his interest in stereos, cars, and power tools — all that guy stuff. Now, I can operate a backpack blower just like the guys, but it doesn't get me very excited.

In a short amount of time, Josh learned Troy's care needs, and became the only other person on the planet (besides me) that could take care of Troy by himself for any length of time.

No one else, not even visiting RNs, could stay alone with Troy. There were so many little details on how things needed to be done to manage his comfort — how to use the suction machine for his saliva, how to clean his nose with q-tips, which was a constant nuisance for him because of allergies. He didn't have the physical strength anymore to blow his nose.

Then there was how to arrange his arms across his lap, adjust his pillows when he lay down, and set up his computer mouse on the floor so he could operate it with his big toe — not to mention lining up his five remote controls for his entertainment system within reach of his foot. He and Josh finally got that down to one or two universal remotes that Troy could operate through his laptop computer.

What made all of this so challenging for others was the difficulty in communication. If Troy had been able to speak, he could have told people what he needed. Instead, he had to rely on me to train them.

Josh did so much more than just taking care of Troy's needs. We came to rely on him for so many things, things that it takes to run a household, from changing the oil in the cars to taking the cat to the vet.

Basically, Josh did many of the things that Troy would have done, had he been able. When I would come home from work, he would often have dinner started.

Now, Josh's cooking is a story in itself. What can I say, but that his heart was in the right place? I still haven't gotten over one of the things he made for us. Sitting on a plate in front of me was wedges of cantaloupe that had been fried in butter in the frying pan, and then sprinkled with the colorful little candies you decorate cupcakes with. Trying to maintain my composure, I politely asked Josh what exactly this was.

"It's one of my grandmother's recipes. She used to make it for us. Isn't it great?" he said, enthusiastically.

When he left the room to take care of Troy, Victoria and I quickly put it down the garbage disposal (sorry, Josh!).

Later, when I checked with his mom about it, I learned that what she had made was fried bananas with brown sugar.

Culinary skills aside, Josh brought an unwavering commitment to us, even though at times that was tremendously challenged. His emotional and physical resources, like mine, were stretched to a level he never knew possible. The difference between Josh and I was that he had the option to give two weeks' notice. He never did...

§

Josh was a support to me beyond words. Just having someone else who had the ability to take Troy in the car was huge!

It was a whole production to drive the chair up the ramp, all the time supporting Troy's head when his neck muscles no longer could. When the chair was at the crest of the ramp, the headrest had to be lowered to clear the door. At that point, the chair had to be taken out of power mode and put into manual.

After losing balance and rolling the chair backwards down the ramp once or twice, I got that part figured out. Still, I would occasionally forget the headrest, in the confusion of everything, and whack his head on the doorway of the van.

Josh was able to help me figure out some tricks to getting the chair in, and maneuvered around to face the front. When Josh did it, he just muscled it into place. I had to do a series of forward and reverse moves in a tight space to get Troy into the front passenger side. Then when we drove, we would use one hand to steer and the other to hold Troy's head up so he could see out.

Computers were a lifeline to Troy. At first, it was a way he could continue to design and write. Later, it became a way he could operate his electronics. But most importantly, the computer became his voice.

With special software designed for the handicapped, he could type what he wanted to say and then have the computer voice-box say it. He formed the words using an onscreen keyboard that scrolled through the letters.

When it got to the letter he wanted, he would press the mouse with his foot to select it. That letter would go into the message box, and then he would search for the next letter.

When he got his message finished, he would hit a command that would cause the voice synthesizer to say whatever he had typed. It took incredible patience and tenacity (maybe a little stubbornness, too), but Troy got good at it.

The program had the ability to create commonly used phrases as well. By choosing a two or three letter code for the phrase he wanted, he could put up a whole phrase at a time.

One of his frequently used codes was HBB, "How's my bride?"

Another was CBB, "Chow! At least for now, baby."

Whenever he wanted Josh, he would use JJJ, "Just joshin' around." Another of Josh's was TTB, "Thank you, bubba!"

There was an art to "spelling" the words so the computer voice would pronounce them the way you wanted.

For instance, Troy got on a kick where he drank Dr. Pepper a lot. To request it, he would use QPP, and the deep robotic voice of the synthesizer would say: "O, wouldn't you want to be ah Pepper too, be ah Pepper! Drink Doctor Pepper! Ohhhh, be ah Pepper, Drink Doctor Pepper!"

He even had his computer speaking French. AAH was "ah, my little mona me."

You could change the computer voice from male to female, child or adult. Now and then, Troy would crack us up by changing the voice to a female — usually when we least expected it, or when things were getting too tense. He liked to pull that on unsuspecting visitors, too. Especially those that would speak louder or extra slow, as if he was hard of hearing, too.

It was amusing to the three of us how often people that came to visit would raise their voices. Even the medical professionals did it.

Usually I would start chuckling, and Josh and Troy would just roll their eyes. Doris, the visiting hospice nurse, would inevitably do it every time she came to visit. She would lean down close to Troy's face and speak to him in a loud, slow voice. Troy and Josh would tease her unmercifully about it. I was usually at work on the days when she would come, but I knew that Troy was one of her favorite patients. She grew to love these two guys.

One day when I was home, Doris broke the news to us that she was retiring. With tears in her eyes, she told us that Troy was one of the most special patients she had ever had. She still came to visit from time to time, even after she retired.

I used to joke with Troy that the patient was supposed to retire in hospice care, not the nurse!

In addition to Josh, we now had help at night, too. During the night, Troy needed medications, suctioning, repositioning, etc. and it became too much for me to do and go to work the next day. We started out with help a couple nights a week, but ultimately went to seven nights.

I started out sleeping in our bed with Troy even though the caregiver was there. I so hated to be away from him. But it was defeating the purpose of my trying to get sleep. So I moved to the couch in the living room, where I was still close by.

Even at that, I knew that when I went to bed, the caregiver might awaken me because Troy needed me for something that they couldn't figure out—not that I could always figure it out, either.

One night when Diane and I were washing Troy's hair, while he was lying in bed, he indicated he wanted to tell us something. Diane would try to spell with him, and then I would try. We could not get what he was trying to tell us. He was getting distressed, and kept looking towards his arm.

After about a million attempts at trying to spell with Troy, Diane finally figured out that his wedding ring had come off when we washed his hands (he had lost so much weight). He didn't want it to be "thrown out with the bath water"!

The night shifts were difficult to fill, too. We were so thankful for Diane when she came along. She is not a nurse by profession, but is certainly a nurturing and loving person by nature. When she learned of our need, our mutual friend, Edna Cooke, had called Diane to see if she would be willing to work for us. Diane had said no to Edna, that it would be too hard for her, both logistically and emotionally. Edna didn't give up. Instead she invited Diane and her husband, Nick, to our home so we could meet. Just a get together to watch a movie on Troy's big screen TV.

Diane told me later that she couldn't keep her eyes off Troy. She felt so much compassion in her heart for him. That night when Troy asked her if she would help, she couldn't say no. She agreed to work one or two nights a week, thinking as we all did, that it would probably be just a few weeks longer that Troy would be with us.

Like Josh, she stuck by us to the end. And that was no small feat!

She drove from Salem, forty-five minutes away, four nights a week, to help us. She had more than her share of driving challenges, from weather conditions to car breakdowns. Not to mention the morning she hit a deer on the way home in the pre-dawn morning light when the deer are typically out.

But she never complained — not even the night she broke two ribs when she fell off the bathroom counter, where she had been standing while cleaning the top of the mirror. She suffered through it, not wanting to have to wake me up, until finally she called her husband to come and get her, and take her to the hospital. Diane was such a giving person; she couldn't stand the thought of being a burden to anyone else.

It continued to amaze and bless us how friends quietly found ways to help. Pastor Keith was consistently visiting or calling us every Wednesday, a spiritual feast when we could no longer get to church. Guy, Troy's co-worker from the county, came from Salem to work on the irrigation system. Roger, Edna's husband, unexpectedly delivered a load of firewood. Dave, Paula's son, brought some kids over from his church and spent the day doing yard work. When the well pump froze and we were without water, Mike came right over and worked outside in the freezing cold until he got it thawed.

My brother Larry continued to work on Troy's computers making adaptations as his needs changed. One time it was more than a new program that needed to be installed—Josh accidentally spilled an entire vase of water on Troy's laptop computer. Patty, our hospice volunteer (and passionate gardener!), brought Troy flowers every week when she came to help, and Troy wanted the vase on the TV tray next to his wheelchair where he could see them. That was also where the laptop computer sat. Josh was forever having to catch that teetering vase after knocking into it on his way by.

After getting over his initial reaction (which maybe took more than a few minutes), Troy got his sense of humor back and teased Josh about his new invention of computer "wetware."

§

By the start of the summer of 1996, Troy's condition seemed to stabilize. The reliability and consistency of Josh and Diane, and the support of hospice, plus the morphine to keep the anxiety levels down were all contributing factors. That and the continual, faithful prayers of friends and untold hundreds, probably thousands, of people we didn't even know. Living with hope was paying off.

After a relentless two years, the progression of the disease seemed to slow down. It had already taken almost everything physically it could have. When we had first moved into the house nine months before, Troy could still speak some, though with great difficulty. Only a few of us could understand him, so when friends would visit they would wait patiently for Troy to formulate his words and then look to me to tell them what he had just said.

That was gone now. He hadn't been able to eat food by mouth for equally as long. That first Thanksgiving after he got his feeding tube, I knew it would be torture for him to have to smell the turkey cooking all day, and not be able to taste it.

So, in crystal glasses set on a beautifully adorned table, I served the family carnation instant breakfast for our Thanksgiving dinner—and tapioca pudding for dessert.

Grandma had brought flowers for Victoria to give to her papa for Thanksgiving. When Victoria took them in and laid them on his lap, she said, "Happy Halloween!"

When she saw the smiles on our faces, she realized something wasn't quite right. She quickly changed it to "Merry Christmas!"

§

We seemed to be out of the crisis mode, at least for now, and more involved in living in the present. With Troy no longer mobile, in some ways it was easier. He no longer was having the terrible falls, and with the feeding tube, we didn't have to live with the constant fear of his choking to death.

Now that we were operating his wheelchair for him (we moved the controls to the back of the chair), I no longer had to worry about him crashing into things, or getting the chair stuck going in circles.

Troy stayed engaged mentally and spent his waking hours working on projects such as landscaping, writing on his computer, and buying me presents.

Josh and he would spend hours pouring over catalogs to find just the right thing for Troy to give me for our anniversary, or Valentine's Day, or my birthday.

For Mother's Day, he ordered me a whole deck full of cedar furniture. I would have said we couldn't afford it, but I was thrilled to get it. I never went shopping for clothes. Not only did I not have the time, I didn't need to. Troy was great at picking stuff out of the Nordstrom catalog and surprising me.

He continued to be a wonderful husband despite the physical limitations, and worked hard at finding ways he could help support me, physically and emotionally.

That year was the first time ever, before or since, that all our Christmas shopping was done and the gifts wrapped by Halloween! He had kept Diane busy at night wrapping the gifts.

We continued to be so thankful and amazed at each season or holiday that Troy continued to be with us. That fall of 1996, Troy's favorite time of year, had many special moments. The sunsets are spectacular that time of year from our deck. It was harvest season for the grapes and hazelnuts, and we could hear the gunshots ring out across the valley at regular intervals as the vineyard owners fired warning shots to keep the birds away from the precious grapes. We have an old orchard of English walnut trees on the property, and I was so excited the first year when the walnuts fell from their husks onto the ground. I made the girls take buckets and go with me to gather up walnuts. They still like to make fun of me and my walnuts.

It was the first season of changing colors on Troy's Japanese maple, planted out front. I wheeled him into the dining room where he could look out on the front courtyard, and see the fountain and the Japanese maple. We spent precious mornings and evenings with fires in the den fireplace, Earl Grey tea, and a new season of Star Trek episodes. We learned to appreciate all the little things that we could.

Now that we had Josh, I felt I could leave Troy for a rare weekend away. My friend, Mary, took me to her condo at Cannon Beach for two nights. I was not much company. I slept almost the entire time. We had brought books and movies, and presto logs for the fireplace, and settled in for a much-needed relaxing weekend. I never knew anyone could sleep so much. The first night I slept for fifteen hours! I got up for a few hours, and went back to bed again for another three hour nap. We did manage to go out for a seafood dinner, but I was in bed again by 9:00 p.m.

Josh said the change in Troy was dramatic while I was gone, and that he greatly improved the day he knew I was coming home.

How do I put into words the connection between Troy and I? The depth of the bond between us? We had truly become a part of each other. Often before he would even start to spell words, I would know what he was going to say. People that witnessed it were awestruck at how I finished his sentences for him after spelling only one or two words. I would just know what he was going to say.

So much was said between us without words. I had mourned the loss of his voice, the loss of the long hours of communication between a husband and wife. I had grieved over not being able to come home from work and talk with my best friend about my day.

However, I gradually discovered that we had something of great value that few others ever get to experience. The loss of the verbal communication was not so devastating as it seemed. Troy and I were learning to communicate spirit to spirit. In a way, it was like how we talk to God — without audible words. My husband and I had discovered a completely new level of communication that is possible between two people that love each other deeply, and take the time to really know and understand each other.

Of course, we had our relationship issues like all marriages do. The previous Valentine's Day, I asked all the nurses and hospice people to stay away so we could have some much needed time alone.

Finding time for just the two of us to be alone was increasingly difficult. Between the day and night nurses, and his mom on the weekends, there was precious little time to ourselves. When it was available, I always had a million other things that needed to be done.

The day started out in anger, and it took quite a bit of the day to get some issues resolved first. Things had been building up like cobwebs in the corner. He was feeling like I had been making all the decisions lately without consulting him. I realized that was true, mostly because it was just faster that way, and time wasn't a luxury I had. And I shared with him that I had been feeling a lack of caring and concern, the protectiveness I was used to getting from him. He recognized that he had been seeing me as more independent, capable of taking care of everything on my own. True, I was capable, but I still wanted his caring and concern!

I remember a co-worker being shocked when I mentioned something Troy and I had argued about.

"You mean you still have arguments, like fights?" she had asked in surprise. She couldn't quite picture that with Troy's illness.

"Of course," I replied. "It's a normal part of marriage. Troy and I will continue to work on our marriage to keep it healthy and to grow as a couple. We'll be working on it to the end."

By the end of the day, we had gotten our hurt feelings resolved. Troy sent me out to the deck, and there, in a clay pot, was a miniature white rose bush. He never ceased to amaze me. No doubt about it — he was definitely "a blessing in disguise."

11
VICTORIA'S VILLAGE

"Children are our most precious flowers."
~Troy Thompson, Landscaper

In other cultures, other times, children would be raised not only by their parents, but also by the whole village. Most of those living in the village were related in one way or another. At times, around our household, it seemed that way for three-year-old Victoria. The lines continued to be a bit fuzzy for her on who was actually "family" and who wasn't.

In her world, many things were out of the ordinary. There were night nurses, day nurses, hospice volunteers who took her to school, weekly pastor visits (who picked her up from school!). Not to mention Grandma every weekend.

Of course, mom and dad were in the picture, too. But when Victoria woke up in the night from a bad dream or not feeling well, she would go find the nurse. She was famous for saying "my tummy has a headache." She seemed to sense that mommy was too exhausted to even comprehend what she needed.

The lights never went out in our house, twenty-four hours a day, and somebody was always up. Doors were never locked because someone was always home. The first time I left the house after Troy was gone, I locked myself out. I had never used the key before!

Victoria became such a bright spot in our crumbling world. Her sweet spirit and young energy, along with the funny things that pre-schoolers say and do, brought laughter and joy into the household. She was a much-needed distraction from the pain and difficulties.

Through her eyes, everything was normal, as it should be. And she seemed to take everything in stride. She was loved very much and always cared for. It was another glimpse of our heavenly father's perspective. That everything is really okay. That he is loving us and caring for us. That he will never turn the lights out...

Troy was her "papa," and he did his best to live up to the role in spite of the overwhelming limitations. One of her "computer codes" was TYO, "Tory, Papa says you must obey." Another was ULW, "love you, you little waskle, you." I think my favorite was the one he used to say "goodnight" to the kids. XXX was "good night, sleep tight, don't let the bed bugs start rumors of a hostile company take over! Papa loves you." The simulated computer voice had a distinct quality to it, and Victoria grew up thinking that was her father's voice.

Their playtime was watching movies together on Troy's computer. She would lie on the bed next to him with her head on his shoulder, and her favorite stuffed lion tucked under her arm.

One day she came home from pre-school saying she had hurt her leg. For the next three days, she limped or crawled around the house, and "needed" to be carried up and down the stairs. There was no apparent injury, but she insisted she was hurt and could not walk. On the third day, we were sitting around the bedroom, our usual gathering place these days when friends or family were around. Troy was working on typing something on his computer. After a minute the computer voice said, "Tory, Papa knows it is very good to tell the truth."

With that, she hopped off the bed. Her leg was "miraculously" healed. All it took was a word from her papa. Amazing what influence fathers have!

Some of the best times for Victoria and I were in the car on the way to school. It was our time alone together each day. She would say the most interesting and insightful (not to mention amusing) things on these morning drives.

I couldn't seem to remember to bring a pen and paper in the car to write them down, but a few of them I will never forget. These little jewels seemed to come out of nowhere.

"Jesus, I'm so proud of you," she said, talking to herself one morning.

When I asked her what she meant, she replied that it was because of the beautiful sparkles he had made. That morning there was frost on the ground, and the sun was making it sparkle like diamonds.

On another morning ride she said, "Mama, when Papa gets better, do you think he will be able to tie my shoes?"

It was so simple, so matter-of-fact. I took a moment to answer, trying to gather my composure and think of something meaningful to say.

"Well," I started out, slowly. "I know your Papa would love to tie your shoes for you." I paused for a moment, and then continued. "But I know, too, that if he never can, God will always provide someone who will tie your shoes for you."

§

I was telling this story the next weekend to our new friend, Barbara. She was another of the huge blessings put into our lives. She had heard about us, and called one day to see how she could help. She became an advocate for keeping prayers flowing for us. She put together a group to specifically pray and work on our growing financial needs.

One day we got a call from our church, saying an usher had found an envelope with our name on it. Inside was $1,000 in cash. No note or explanation, just ten $100 bills.

On another occasion, a pastor from a church in Newberg whom we had never met paid us a visit. He brought with him $500 from someone in his congregation. Unknown to us, his church had been praying for us, and this particular couple had felt moved to help in this way.

As I was telling the story to Barbara about "tying shoes," her mouth dropped open, and she let out a little scream.

She rushed out to her car, and came back with a package.

"I was saving this to give to Victoria for Christmas," she said excitedly. "But, I think we should give it to her now."

Barbara helped Victoria open the package. Inside was a beautiful book entitled *Does God Know How to Tie Shoes?*

§

Yes, Victoria had assumed her father's role as a "blessing in disguise." We had planned to name this child Troy if she had been a boy. Instead, we named her Tory as a nickname for Victoria. Her name, and her spirit, became increasingly significant as time went on. Victoria — victorious! Just like her papa…

12
"BUT THEY DON'T KNOW TROY!"

Josh and I made a pact. Standing in the kitchen, dishtowel over his shoulder, he told me that no matter what anyone said, or tried to predict, we were going to keep a positive attitude.

Even when the prognosis was frightening, we were always to believe that Troy wasn't going anywhere a day sooner than God had planned.

We promised each other that if one of us got down, the other would kick their rear!

It seemed like every time Troy and I came back from a doctor's visit, I would have to work hard at not starting to panic. Every time I would try to close the door on the monster, it would come in through the window.

"What do they know?" Josh would say. "They don't know Troy!"

Josh was right about that! Troy's fighting spirit and will to live, along with his sense of humor, and most importantly his faith, kept him with us far beyond what the doctors predicted.

Weeks turned into months, and still Josh continued to work for us as Troy continued to live. That summer, Josh and Troy went on many outings in the van, usually to electronics or video stores. On several occasions, they surprised me and stopped by my office. Josh would hop out of the van and run in with a bouquet of roses, usually two red with one white — the red roses represented me and Troy and the white one symbolized Christ as the center of our marriage.

That fall, on October 30, 1996, the hospice nurse heard "rubs" in all four places on Troy's lungs. This was the first time that had ever happened.

I tried not to panic, but we both knew that his lungs were the critical component to keeping him alive.

We called Dr. Edwards, Troy's pulmonologist, who came over as soon as he could the next day, even though it was a Sunday. He reassured us that Troy's upper air passages were still good. The noises were mostly in the lower back, something he would keep an eye on.

It had been a year or so since we had seen Dr. Edwards, during which time he had retired from his practice at OHSU. Dr. Edwards was thrilled — and amazed — to see that Troy was still alive and doing so well.

§

By the next spring, the trips in the van had all but stopped. Troy's neck muscles had grown so weak he could not hold his head up at all. Going over the slightest bump with the wheelchair was jarring to his head and neck.

It was difficult when visitors came because Troy could no longer hold his head up to see them. His only view was of his lap. He began spending more and more time in bed. It was easier on his neck than having his head hanging there like a dead weight. It also meant he could look at people when he communicated with them. The new "post" for those of us taking care of Troy was a small swivel stool next to the bed. We would sit there for hours at a time, spelling words with him.

Even with the computer set up next to his bed, which he operated with his big toe, there were times when he was too tired.

At these times, we would use a spelling chart to communicate. One of the tricks to spelling with Troy was writing down each letter as we figured it out. Otherwise, we would get several letters stringing together, and then forget the first one or two, and have to start over again. (We learned to keep a pad of paper and pencil by the bed!)

Another trick was being able to spell! Spelling was not necessarily one of Troy's strong suits. As happened on many occasions, we were working on a word one evening that I was having trouble figuring out. So far he had spelled:

C A L S T E R F O I C

When I couldn't figure out what the word was, he switched gears and spelled "small place." Oh well. I guess claustrophobic is not a word too many people know how to spell!

March 14, 1997 marked our fifth wedding anniversary and the one-year anniversary of Josh's employment with us. Amazing!

At the end of March, Dr. Johnston came over for a home visit. Troy hadn't seen her since November of 1995, a year and a half ago. We kept in touch by phone, but the visits to OHSU had become too difficult. Besides, there was not a lot the doctor could do at that point. She answered any questions we had, and prescribed medications, but we had long since stopped trying to measure his progression. Her medical notes, which I later read, said:

"His survival in the past year is unexpected, given the degree of respiratory impairment and severe progression of the disease. I, therefore, find it difficult to prognosticate."

§

The next month Troy's dad, Jerry, came from Arizona for another visit. While he was here this time, he brought Troy's grandmother over to the house. It was her 94th birthday, and she had not seen Troy since the illness. She, too, was in a wheelchair, and Jerry borrowed our van to bring her to the house for a visit.

Troy got out of bed for the occasion, and I wheeled him into the den. His grandma wanted her wheelchair right up next to his so she could hold his hand.

It was quite a moving sight, these two side by side in their wheelchairs. Grandmother sat hunched over in hers, covered by a hand-knit blue and white afghan. She had insisted that her daughter do her makeup before Troy came in to see her. Her thinning white hair was combed, and lipstick and rouge applied.

She didn't say anything when she saw Troy. She just reached her gnarled, age-spotted hand across to cover Troy's smooth, limp hand. Troy's head lay so far forward his chin touched his chest. Wearing a t-shirt, his exposed arms were as thin as hers.

Victoria was excited to discover she had another grandma that she had not known about. She would go over to her wheelchair and talk to her, and pat her arm. Grandmother, at 94, was hard of hearing, so after Victoria would talk to her, she would come over to me and say, "Why's her not talking to me?"

She passed away quietly that next December. Troy's eyes filled with tears when I gave him the news. He asked me if I would mind going to the funeral and taking flowers. Victoria and I went, even though she didn't really understand what it was all about. For years afterward, Victoria would still talk about her grandmother, the one that "can't walk."

§

After several months of sleeping on the couch, I made the decision to sleep in a real bed, and moved downstairs to a spare room. These kinds of decisions were difficult. Emotionally, it was one step further away from Troy. Practically speaking, it brought up the question of wondering if it was worth the trouble of buying a bed and setting up a bedroom, not knowing how much longer he would be with us.

My neck and shoulder muscles were constantly in pain from lifting Troy and the awkward position of bending over his bed, closely watching his eyebrows as we painstakingly spelled word after word. Sleeping on the couch wasn't helping, either.

We had started using a baby monitor to listen for Troy when we were not in the room. After the move downstairs, the night caregiver would bring the baby monitor downstairs at 6:00 a.m. to the room where I was sleeping. They would wake me up so I could listen for the groans that Troy would make, indicating he needed something. Troy was so dependent on others. I know that monitor made him nervous. Every now and then one of us would forget to turn it on, or the batteries would run out while I was outside. It was so distressing for him to try to get our attention, and have no one come.

One of the short-lived night caregivers had trouble staying awake. A couple of times I awoke suddenly during the night, and went upstairs to see if everything was okay. It was that same kind of instinct that causes a mother to wake up, even before her baby cries. I found Troy all stressed out, and the nurse snoring away in a chair. We didn't keep her very long.

Even though I was in a total state of exhaustion, sleep wouldn't always come. Many nights I lay there, too tired to sleep. I prayed for the escape of sleep, to get away from this huge ache inside of longing for Troy. Even though he was still here, upstairs, I missed him so much.

I don't know which was worse — knowing he was upstairs and not being able to be with him, or the enormous dread that would sweep over me as I imagined the dark days ahead when he would be gone.

On Easter, we had one of those rare few hours alone together. It wasn't planned that way. But a huge windstorm came through and knocked the power out.

Family and friends that were planning to come over delayed until later in the day, waiting to see if we would get our electricity back. Troy was having a tough time emotionally.

Through tears he spelled out, "All I want is to be able to walk through the garden with you."

Yes, my dear husband. One day we will...

§

Yet another June came and went. I was asked to speak at the annual ALS symposium held at OHSU, on the topic of communication. Dr. Johnston had used Troy's example many times in talking to different doctors. His experience was uncharted ground, for a hospice patient to be on morphine for such an extended period of time, and with these surprising results.

Afterward, several doctors and medical professionals came up to me, having heard about Troy. Their comments encouraged me that something extraordinary was going on. And the hope continued.

I remember the day we first met Kenny. Like Troy, Kenny had been afflicted with ALS, this worst of all diseases, at a young age. I met Kenny at the ALS symposium, and he asked if he could come over and meet my husband.

Arrangements were made, and Kenny came to the house with his caregiver. Unlike Troy, Kenny's disease was progressing unusually slowly. Even though he had been suffering from the disease for a longer period of time, he could still walk with assistance, as well as speak in a slurred sort of way. He sat in a chair next to Troy's bed, and earnestly asked Troy what advice he could give him on how to spend these limited number of days left of his life.

It was obvious from the difference in their physical conditions that Troy's days would be a lot fewer than Kenny's.

Did Troy have any regrets? Was there anything that he would do differently?

Troy was having difficulty answering with the extremely emotional situation of these two men, who shared a disease that was cutting short their lives.

I remember Troy telling Kenny to love his family, to read the Bible, to give his life to the Lord.

I'll never forget when Kenny said, "I want what you have. I want a marriage like yours." With a twinkle in his eye, he said he wasn't going to give up.

And he didn't! A few months later, Kenny fell in love and married his caregiver, Melanie. They even had a baby daughter!

§

Troy's dad visited again for Father's Day, and again we went through the string of June birthdays. This year, 1997, was Holly's turn to graduate from high school. We had a big barbecue for her at the house. Later, in a quiet moment with just the girls and Josh (now considered part of the family), we asked Holly to come into the bedroom where Troy was.

Lying beside Troy was a stuffed bear wearing a graduation cap and gown, and an envelope tucked under its arm. In the envelope were the keys to the 1969 Volkswagen Fastback we had gotten Holly for graduation.

Troy beamed at her squeal of delight. He loved giving surprises.

Josh took a much-needed vacation, and went to Missouri for a week to visit relatives. I have to admit, both Troy and I were nervous at the thought of Josh being so far away. We had come to depend so much on him.

Since working for us, Josh had moved to Newberg to be closer, and there were times that I would have to call him to come back when I needed his help. It could be any number of things, from difficulty breathing to muscle cramps to bowel problems. There were some of these times that it took both of us to handle it.

But Josh desperately needed a break. He was starting to have shoulder and back problems, too. Every one of us that took care of Troy for any length of time had back injuries.

Josh, Diane, and Colby (another night caregiver) all had to take time off when they hurt their back. It would always cause major anxiety for us trying to fill the gap, and not knowing when they would be able to come back, but somehow we got through.

During one of these times when I was taking care of Troy more than usual, we worked on a project of gathering together all his poetry. Over the years, Troy had written many poems, a hobby he enjoyed that was second only to his love of black and white photography, which grace the walls of our den.

I sat and read to him poem after poem. The more I read, the more poetry I found that had been written to old girlfriends. After awhile, I was getting a little tired of reading these, and gave him a bad time about it. He typed on his computer: "Van Gogh—did he have to go through this?" Troy's sense of humor was always ready to leap into play.

13
POINT MAN AND REAR GUARD

"Your righteousness will go before you, and the glory of the Lord
will be your rear guard."
(Isaiah 58:8)

At first, I was merely somewhat amused when I looked at the treasured G.I. Joe that had survived many a battle put on by seven-year-old Troy and friends.

Joe, now pushing twenty-nine years, lived in a green wooden box, along with his battle gear. Troy would have ten-year-old Michelle dress him up in his dress whites or his camouflage fatigues and set on top of the computer where Troy could see him from his bed.

That summer, for Troy's 36th birthday, his mom gave him a new, limited edition of G.I. Joe. That was only the beginning. Every day when I would come through the door from work, there would be that twinkle in his eye and sheepish grin. He and Josh tried to distract me from the growing display of Joes.

As the new GI Joes continued to arrive, boxes starting piling up around the bedroom. Soon they were taking over the walk-in closet, too.

With Josh's help, Troy would give detailed instructions, spelled out on his computer, about how these soldiers were to be displayed. They were placed in battle ready positions on shelves, in Troy's line of sight.

As finances were being squeezed with the enormous medical expenses we were facing, I found myself getting slightly irritated. These Joes did not come cheap!

"Don't worry, honey, they're collectibles! They'll be worth a lot someday," Troy tried to reassure me. What was he thinking? None of us would be able to part with a single one of those Joes!

Then one evening something happened that I will never forget. It was one of those times you just know God is speaking to you.

During a powerful prayer time when a small group of us were gathered around the bed, God revealed to me an awesome glimpse of his perspective from above.

These poised and battle ready figures were a symbolic, yet tangible message for us. We were at war! Frontline, heat of the battle, point men fighting in a full-scale war. Not only against the horrible disease, but also against death itself.

In addition to the faithful few God put on the frontlines with us, he raised up an entire army to work behind the battle lines. Friends and churches all over the world were standing behind us as support troops. Just when we would think we couldn't go another day, fresh troops would be sent in.

Certainly some days were quieter than others as the enemy called death was strategizing and re-loading weapons. At other times, the bullets came in rapid-fire succession…

But God promises to go before us, and behind us.

§

One night during a particularly challenging time, Troy spelled out to me that he wished the end would come. It was the first time he had ever said that. Then he added, "But I don't want to leave you."

On one other occasion that I recall, he was close to defeat. Mary Beth, the woman who had lost her husband to ALS and become a close friend of ours, came by for a visit. Troy was really down. She remembers trying to cheer him up, but he just looked away.

"Is there anything I can do?" she asked, concerned.

It took awhile for her to figure out what Troy was trying to say.

"Did you just say what I think you said?" she asked. "Did you say it's time to get Kevorkian?"

Troy raised his eyebrows with a yes.

"You don't mean that!" she said. "I know what you think of that dirty dog!"

Dr. Kevorkian had become world famous for his methods of euthanasia in assisting people to die. She knew that Troy despised what this man was doing.

Troy just rolled his eyes. He didn't really mean what he was saying. It was his way of communicating that it was one of those low points when he felt like giving up. No matter how strong you are, how strong your beliefs, those times come. We're only human.

Even though the progression had slowed down, there seemed to consistently be new challenges. Bedsores became a problem, not only on his tailbone, but also on his cheekbone from having his head always turned on the same side. It was the only way he was comfortable.

Rosemary, one of our first night caregivers, came up with what we later called the "doughnut pillows." She sewed together a circle of soft fabric, about 8 inches across, with a hole in the center. She stuffed it with a soft pillow stuffing. Placed under the side of his face that he lay on, they helped to keep his head up off his cheekbone.

Another unexpected challenge was his teeth. He started clenching his jaw, uncontrollably, and was literally breaking off his teeth and fillings. He hated feeling those little particles in his mouth that he was afraid of choking on, and yet it was extremely difficult for us to get inside his mouth and find them.

On Thanksgiving, I spent all morning trying to swab out his mouth without gagging him. One of his front teeth had become so loose that I ended up pulling it out with my bare hands. I still shake my head in amazement at what crazy things I did for my husband!

All of us have those days or weeks when everything seems to be falling apart. But coupled with this horrendous disease, there were days that I didn't know how we were going to make it. In one of those weeks, Holly came down with mono, the furnace went out, our savings account was nearly drained, the cat was missing, and Troy came down with a miserable sinus infection.

Thank God for the support troops. As difficult as it was for us, it was also extremely difficult for those that faithfully came alongside us. But they didn't let on. They kept their fears to themselves, and did their grieving away from the house.

Pastor Keith would later share with me what some of his visits were like from his perspective. He looked forward to our time together, and at the same time, he had a certain dread. He knew that even in the short time between visits there would be some new change, something else that we would be faced with.

Many times when he left, he would cry out to God on the drive home, "Lord, I don't know how they can handle much more. I don't know if they can make it if one more thing happens, let alone just get through this."

But, as Keith would say, the Lord came through, often at 11:59, and multiplied the five loaves into thousands.

An example was our financial situation. Several things happened, sometimes miraculously, to assure that we always had what we needed. For instance, just prior to getting Troy's diagnosis, we had doubled his life insurance. The approval was given only days before we learned that there may be something worse than a strained muscle in Troy's back.

Then at a point when our money was running out, we discovered that because Troy had been diagnosed as having less than a year to live, we were able to draw on that policy for up to 80% of its value. That alone saved us from having to liquidate our assets in order to pay for the approximately $40,000 per year out of pocket that wasn't covered by insurance. Part of that was the caregiver salaries that exceeded the limit paid for by insurance, plus the many vitamins and supplements (and millions of q-tips!) that weren't covered.

When it came to our medical insurance, that was another miracle. As more and more time went by, we found ourselves in a situation where Troy's medical insurance through his former employer was going to run out. Without going into all the insurance jargon, and Oregon law, let me just say that the generous policy that we had was ending, and we were soon to be eligible for Medicare.

The problem was that Medicare didn't have the benefits we had for caregiver salaries that our insurance had been willing to cover. Sitting at the kitchen table, I had no idea what we were going to do. The fear was rising up and threatening to turn into full-blown despair. I did the one thing I knew to do—I prayed. I picked up the phone and made yet another call to the state of Oregon. But this time I got a different answer.

That day, just the right person answered my call and I will never forget how she graciously helped me. After listening to my explanation of what was going on, she did some extra digging and discovered a brand new law regarding "portability insurance" that had just gone into effect the month before. It was so new and obscure that the insurance companies didn't even know about it. I got a written copy of the law from the state and provided it to our insurance company. With that, we were able to stay on our private insurance in addition to Medicare.

The amazing thing about all of this was the timing. If I had discovered this a couple months later, our "cobra insurance" period would have run out and the timing would have been too late for us, even with this law.

As a songwriter said, if I had a thousand years, I would still run out of time to tell the world what an awesome God we have.

§

In July of 1997, the Oregonian contacted us about doing a story on death and dying. They had heard about Troy, and his fight for life against the odds. The story was to profile five different terminally ill people, and their attitudes towards dying. We agreed to do the story.

Over the next two months, we spent several hours with Mark O'Keefe, the Oregonian reporter doing the series. In addition to Mark, there were three different days of photo shoots with Michael Lloyd, a staff photographer. I invited both of them to come to Troy's birthday celebration in August where they might pick up more pieces to the story from friends and family.

What a celebration it turned out to be! Eighty-five people came to see Troy and marvel at his amazing strength and courage. It was not easy for everyone. As Dean, one of my sales agents, said, "Frankly, I was quite nervous about seeing him. It's just so hard. But when I saw him smile, I knew it was okay! He's in there, and I know he's okay."

Nancy, who also worked for me at the time, put it this way: "I admired your courage to do the party. That was just what everybody needed. Denny (her husband) was speechless."

"Why didn't you tell me more about what was happening to Troy?" he asked.

"Because you wouldn't have understood until you experienced it," she told her husband. She went on to say that it was wonderful to celebrate Troy's birthday with him, but "he is the one who gave each of us a gift...of understanding and inspiration."

For a few, it was the first time they had seen Troy since the illness. It's sad how some just cannot deal with it, and end up staying away.

I learned that it is not because they don't care. It's that they care so much...but don't know how to face it. In actuality, what happened for several friends took them by surprise.

Seeing the way Troy looked was difficult for sure, but surprisingly inspiring. Because of Troy's contagious smile and courage, they found it to be a rewarding experience.

Many expressed that they would be back — and were wishing they had come sooner.

One of those was Dort (short for Dorothy), Troy's 84-year-old "adopted" grandmother. Until now, she couldn't bring herself to see Troy. We were surprised and overjoyed to learn that she was coming to the party.

I know several people felt that they were being given a chance to see Troy one last time, and they did not want to have regrets later.

When Dort came into the bedroom, and leaned down and kissed Troy on the cheek, we all lost it. I took a tissue and wiped Troy's eyes.

Dort started going on and on about when Troy was just a little boy. The more she talked, the more she and Troy cried. I tried to lighten up the conversation, and steer her into the other room.

Finally, she let Mom take her into the kitchen for some food. But the minute she got her food, she insisted on bringing her plate and a chair, so she could sit right next to the bed close to Troy.

Everything about that day was wonderful. But as I will never stop saying, it is the friends and support that continues to amaze and bless me. Patty, our hospice volunteer and gardener extraordinaire, did stunning bouquets of flowers. Jill, a long time friend of Troy's, catered all the food.

Josh did valet parking. Actually, it was the only thing I could think of to get him out of the house. When I arrived home from work just a half hour before guests were to arrive, he was running around the house in a panic at all these people coming over.

Kathy Goeddel, another ALS widow like Mary Beth, had arranged for a professional magician to come for entertainment. As it turned out, the magician was not only entertaining, especially for all the kids, but he was so touched by the whole thing that he would not accept payment.

Troy got tons of touching cards and presents, including the GI Joe from his Mom that started the collection, and a full size cardboard statue of Darth Vader from Star Wars (brought by Mary Beth). One of the most touching was a bonsai tree brought by Ted Nelson, Troy's former boss. He and Troy shared the common interest of bonsais. They had loved to work on their hobby together, usually one night a week after work, and would spend hours clipping, wiring, and shaping these little miniature trees. They had a friendly competition going, trying to out-do one another. For Troy's birthday, Ted brought him his most prized bonsai. Troy was deeply moved. And as Ted would later tell the story…

"As I gave Troy my favorite bonsai tree, I saw that twinkle in his eye. Two hours later, I walked out of their house very humbled. And I understood. Troy surprised me by giving me his favorite bonsai. Which, coincidentally, was about three times the size and four times as good as my puny specimen. As usual, Troy out-did me one more time."

§

While Michael was busy shooting photographs, Mark, the reporter, was going from room to room with his notepad and pen, interviewing people. After spending a fair amount of time with these guys, we became friends.

A year or so later when I got back in touch with Michael about getting copies of the photos, he shared with me how Troy had affected his life in a personal way.

While working with power tools in his garage on a woodworking project, he had cut off the ends of several fingers. For a photographer, it was devastating.

But he remembered what Troy had gone through, and how he had handled it with such a positive attitude. Michael took the attitude that things could have been a lot worse, and was thankful for what he still had to live for.

A few weeks after the party, Mark came back and read us the final draft on the story. It was highly unusual for the Oregonian to allow this, but they compassionately granted our request. We didn't want any surprises or misquotes in our fragile emotional state.

While reading it to us, Mark had to stop more than once, and the three of us cried together. When he finished, he looked at us with hopeful anticipation.

"Well, what do you think?" he asked eagerly.

"It is absolutely wonderful, Mark," I replied. "You have done an amazing job."

Troy's smile voiced the same sentiment.

We knew when Mark left that day, final draft in hand, that our little world was about to change. Our story was going public. But we had no idea how far-reaching that would be. We put our trust in God to go before us…and behind us.

14
IN THE SPOTLIGHT

"Every great book has been written with the author's blood."[1]

Standing in the kitchen at 6:30 a.m., I poured myself a cup of coffee. Troy was sleeping, and Diane had just left. It was Tuesday, Sept. 30, 1997, the day the article about Troy was to run in the Oregonian. The four-day series had started on Sunday with an overview of the five people being interviewed.

We really hadn't known anything about the format, and I was surprised when I picked up the Sunday Oregonian and saw Troy's smiling face on page 18 of the front section.

The full page was titled "Facing Death" and had photos of five terminally ill people, ranging in age from 36 to 84—Troy was the youngest. Two had cancer, one had AIDS, and the other had a breathing disorder.

Under Troy's photo the caption read:

Troy Thompson, Age 36, Lou Gehrig's Disease

Troy, who is paralyzed, can no longer speak. His wife, Marilyn Thompson, said this for him: "You go through the

---

[1] Cowman, Lettie B. *Streams in the Desert* (Grand Rapids: Zondervan, 1997), p. 43.

whys. You go through the anger. But I guess that when we see the growth that has taken place…it's extraordinary. Troy has had more impact on people disabled than he would have had if he were healthy."

The basis for the series was the controversy surrounding doctor-assisted suicide in Oregon. The voters in Oregon had passed a ballot measure in 1994, becoming the first state in the country to sanction doctor-assisted suicide.

Now, three years later, Oregonians were being asked to consider Ballot Measure 51, a referendum that would repeal this law.

With one month to go before the November elections, the Oregonian was running this series, showing the different sides of the highly controversial and emotionally charged issue.

Of the five people featured in the series, some were for and some against doctor-assisted suicide.

Troy was very clear on his position.

He was against it.

Interestingly, it was 1994 when the law passed. I have to admit, I was so caught up in life…my new marriage, a new baby… that I really hadn't paid much attention to the issue.

I don't recall Troy and I ever discussing it prior to the election that year. Not until we were having coffee and reading the morning paper in the living room of the Columbia Gorge Hotel, a classic old hotel overlooking the Columbia River. We had gone up there for a weekend away shortly after getting the diagnosis. It's a romantic setting with the majestic river below on one side, and beautiful gardens on the other. It is such a beautiful spot, we had considered having our wedding there.

This weekend was another one of those almost desperate attempts to try to have whatever time we could as a couple before Troy became too sick.

In the Oregonian newspaper that particular Sunday morning was front-page news about the doctor-assisted suicide ballot measure in the upcoming May elections.

With Troy's new status as "terminally ill," the article caught our attention. We were struck by the timing of this issue and Troy's situation. We both looked at each other and knew that in some way, some time, Troy was going to be playing a role. That thought went on a back burner until three years later when Mark O'Keefe from the Oregonian called us to do the story.

§

With coffee cup in hand, and still in my bathrobe, I hopped in the car to go retrieve the morning paper. I was hopeful that at this early hour none of the neighbors would be out to see me still in my "morning attire."

I drove quickly to the bottom of the long driveway. Looking both directions, the coast was clear, and I jumped out and grabbed the paper out of the box. My heart was pounding as I set the paper on the seat next to me. I didn't even want to look at it until I was back in the sanctuary of our home.

Holding my breath, I carefully laid the paper out on the kitchen table. I gasped aloud when I saw my photo on the front page! There I was, standing outside our open bedroom door with Josh and Troy in the background. The photo portrayed me as if in a moment of contemplation about our lives. (But did he really have to use a side view?! Oh well, no time for vanity now!)

The article was titled "One Man's Dying," and the caption under my photo read:

"When Marilyn Thompson learned her husband had an incurable, terminal disease that would leave him paralyzed and speechless, she resolved to make the most of whatever time they had left."

I quickly started to read, then stopped when I saw that the article was going to continue on page A6.

Opening the paper, I was flabbergasted! Not only did the article continue, it covered three more full pages, covered in photos!

There were photos with Victoria showing her papa a birthday card from his party, one with Josh leaning over Troy and doing arm stretches, one with his mom sitting on our "stool" and sharing a laugh with Troy.

There was one with his best friends from West Linn High School sitting around the bed with him, and another showing a close-up of his foot operating the computer mouse with his big toe.

By now, I was shaking with disbelief at the magnitude of the article. I pulled out a chair and sat down. I sat there with both hands wrapped around my coffee cup, taking sips of coffee and staring at all those photos of our bedroom, our life. No sound was coming over the monitor from Troy's room so I slowly turned back to the front page and started reading from the beginning…

§

Going to work that day was difficult. I really just wanted to go somewhere and hide. Anyone who knows me will tell you that I am a particularly private person. This was probably especially true at work. As the manager of the office, I generally kept my private life separate from work.

I sat in my car for a few minutes, and finally got up the courage to go in. This was way out of my comfort zone!

The first two people to greet me in the morning are always my secretary and receptionist. When I walked in, both had obviously been crying. One was still wiping her eyes with tissue, the newspaper still spread out in front of her on the desk.

One by one, throughout the day, the salespeople would stop by my office, and cry, and tell me how moved they were by the story. Most people didn't know our story in this kind of detail, and were extremely moved.

Tom, one of my sales staff, described himself that morning reading the newspaper at the breakfast table:

"I couldn't stop crying into my cereal as I read the story. I didn't move from the table for almost forty-five minutes. After that I didn't want to go to work, but then I realized that was hogwash. I am so lucky just to be able to go to work and have a normal day."

Another sales agent, Steve, could barely get his words out through his tears (he always joked about being an emotional Irishman).

"Powerful, powerful," was all he could manage to say when he sat down in my office. When I asked him what message came through for him he managed to say, "Never, never, never give up."

"Troy will like that," I said.

§

It was weird going places that day and seeing my picture on the front page of the newspaper everywhere I went. Standing next to me in line at Starbucks was a guy reading the article! Troy always had to have Starbuck's cappuccinos, even though it was usually out of our way. Josh and I would take turns going to get them. And we couldn't get away with a substitute. I tried. More than once. I mean, how can he really tell? It goes through his feeding tube, for heaven's sake!

Anyway, I kept looking away, hoping this guy wouldn't recognize me. (I should have brought some of those Jack Nicholson dark glasses!) On the table was another copy of the paper with my photo. And more in the newsstands. I couldn't get out of there fast enough.

The phone rang all day at the office and at home. Josh and Troy called me several times with updates on the volume of emails and phone calls that were coming to the house. At work, the calls and emails were from people I knew.

But the big surprise was at home. So many calls and notes were from total strangers. Mark had included our email address in the article, but not our phone number or address. I guess people just looked it up, because the phone never stopped ringing until almost ten o'clock that night.

Some of the calls and letters that came were from people who had a family member with ALS. Some were from people thanking us for sharing our inspiring story. Some were to offer prayer support. And some were from old friends and acquaintances of mine or Troy's that recognized us. Of course, one or two of them were an old girlfriend of Troy's. But hey, it was okay. They were all very compassionate.

I went to bed exhausted that night from all the emotion and sheer adrenaline. I have always taught my salespeople that when we get out of our comfort zone, and do the things that are often the most difficult — that is when the real growth happens. So true.

Over the next several days, the emails and letters kept coming. The first day alone we got over two hundred e-mails. We even received emails and letters from different parts of the country as Oregonians passed the article along to family and friends.

In addition to the many heartfelt "thank-you for sharing your story and changing my life" letters, the suggestions of various therapies to try, and the many wonderful prayers, we also received an offer to help with maintaining Troy's bonsais (which Troy accepted), a pair of "hand-fed cockatiels" (which he didn't accept), and financial donations.

The Oregonian was also flooded with phone calls and emails. Mark shared that it was one of the biggest responses they had ever had. It was a proud moment for all of us a few months later when Mark was nominated for a national award for that series on "Death and Dying."

Angie, Tom's wife, also worked for me. Her mom taught fourth grade and read the article to her class. Half way through, concerned about their attention span, she stopped and asked the kids if they wanted her to keep going. This was a long article for nine-year-olds to sit through. She looked up from her reading to see the room full of wide-eyed little faces that all nodded in unison. It was clear they were listening. She had the kids write letters to us and share their feelings. One of the little boys wrote:

Dear Troy and Marilyn,

I was touched by the story in the newspaper. It will give me strength and courage when I think about the story, especially if I ever get a disease like you have, Troy. I will look up to you whenever I'm hurt. I hope Troy will live a lot longer than the doctors expect. I bet you will because of your strength and courage. I will pray for you every day. I hope you like my letter.

Jack
4th Grader

Another particular favorite was from Clarence Nagel, a ninety-one-year-old man (hey, another Clarence!). He wrote us several hand-written letters, each one multiple pages long. With each letter, he would include a check to help with costs, which I suspect that he probably couldn't afford to be giving. He gave long dissertations on the value of vitamins and supplements to treat diseases, a theory to which we also subscribed.

Among the "support troops" who arrived in our life were Karen and Ellen, who educated us further on nutrition and supplementation. With their help, we changed Troy's diet from the doctor prescribed liquid food known as "Jevity" (or Ensure) and started using a juicer to give Troy "real food." We juiced everything from raw potatoes to beets to watermelon.

Although it was a lot more work, the healthier diet, along with lots of different minerals and vitamins, allowed us to take Troy off over half of the prescription medicines. His skin color and circulation improved. His bedsores almost completely disappeared. We believe this was one of the components that added to his longevity.

Among the emails was one from Paul Linnman, news anchor at KATU in Portland, who wrote Troy an awesome letter. In part, it read:

"Troy, let me just say flat out, you are my new hero! I was blown away by Mark O'Keefe's story on you today in the Oregonian. I basically spend my days visiting with and interviewing inspirational story subjects, but I'll put you ahead of all of them. (It's quite a list, too. I've met 1,027 great people in "The Spirit of the Northwest" series alone.)

...I honestly believe that we need heroes, role models. They help us get through some pretty bleak days. But, unfortunately, most of us — especially the kids — choose the wrong ones. Today, you must believe that you are a hero, a real life role model. Worthy of emulation, as a man, a husband, father and Christian, to untold thousands who only came to hear your story in the Oregonian for the very first time. Troy, most of us couldn't accomplish that in ten lifetimes..."

The whole experience was remarkable. All the moving stories of how Troy's example was touching and changing so many lives served to boost his spirits and energy beyond anything we could have done. His hope and will to live grew even stronger.

§

A couple weeks later Mark O'Keefe called.

"Have you been getting all the emails I'm forwarding to you?" he asked. "Pretty amazing stuff!"

"I have been getting lots of requests from other papers and reporters wanting to get in touch with you," he continued. "I've tried to shield you from most of them, but there was one today that sounded like something you may want to consider."

He went on to tell us about a major Japanese television network, NHK, who had contacted him, asking if he thought we would be willing to do an interview.

The interest in the whole issue of doctor-assisted suicide and Oregon's law was drawing international attention.

The Los Angeles bureau for NHK was in Portland to cover the story during the election, and they wanted to feature our family in their newscast.

Troy was excited because he knew the television network. He watched it on cable TV occasionally, even though it was all in Japanese, because he enjoyed catching glimpses of Japanese gardens. We agreed to the interview.

They came on Wednesday, my day at home with Troy. It was a rainy, blustery day. They arrived in shiny black sedans. Five men were standing politely at the door when I opened it. A sharply dressed man named Yoshi, the youngest in the group (and obviously from Los Angeles), spoke English and handled the introductions. Besides Yoshi, who was the field producer, there was the camera operator and Mr. Suzuki, the bureau chief. The other two men, dressed in dark suits, didn't speak English.

I invited them to come in to the bedroom where Troy was. They set up the cameras, and requested that we just go about our normal life as they filmed. One man went all around shooting pictures of the inside of the house, the family photos, Troy's bonsais, and then went outside and took even more pictures!

"You mean you want me to act normal with these cameras on us?" I joked.

Other than the camera operator, the others stood politely off to the side, not saying a word. After several minutes of this, I asked again if this was what they wanted. "Isn't this getting a little boring?" I asked with a smile. All I was doing so far was giving Troy his medications, helping him get his email up on the computer, and helping him spell an occasional sentence.

"No, you're doing just fine," was the reply.

After about forty-five minutes of this, they asked Troy if he would give, in his own words, his opinion on physician-assisted suicide.

"Take as long as you need," they told him.

Troy started typing on his computer with his toe. By this point, it was an extremely slow process. His program would put up the alphabet and go through the rows. When it got to the row with the letter he wanted, he would push down on the clicker with his toe.

The problem now was that his toe would not react fast enough to the signal from his brain. He would miss the row over and over. Finally, when he would get the right row, the cursor would move across the row to the letters in that row.

If he missed the letter, which happened most of the time, he would have to start all over again choosing the row. It was painful to watch as he struggled. But he wanted to do this himself.

I left the room to go talk to Holly and Yoshi in the kitchen while Troy worked on the computer. The plan, Yoshi told me, was to run the story on their prime time news in Japan. It would be seen by thousands of people — maybe over a million.

The whirring and beeping sounds that Troy's program makes stopped. I went in to see if he was done. He looked upset.

One of the men explained to me that he had gotten a few words on the screen and then it all disappeared. Seeing it was too much for Troy to have to try to do this with the added pressure of an audience, I offered to spell with him. He gratefully agreed, and I sat next to the bed and spelled with him, letter by letter, writing each one down as we went.

When we finished I asked Troy, just to be sure. I showed him what was written on the paper.

"Is this what you want to say as your answer to why you are opposed to doctor-assisted suicide?"

His eyebrows up gave me a yes.

I paused and looked at the men. Then I looked into the camera and said, "My husband said 'God doesn't make mistakes, we do. God is the author and finisher of our lives.'"

§

Another interview we agreed to do was for a major newspaper in Portugal, Spain. This time it was just two men that came to the house, arriving early one evening. One was a photographer, and one was the reporter.

The interesting thing to me was how moved they both were from meeting Troy and spending time with us. I guess it was true what the one woman had said from the party; that you really have to experience it to understand what it was like at our house on the hill in Newberg, Oregon.

I liked the way one woman described it in her letter to the Oregonian. She called it a "true love story."

Yes, it was a love story. It was a story about the love of friends…and the love of strangers.

It was a love between a man and a woman, husband and wife, our lives and dreams torn apart by a devastating disease, and rebuilt into a castle of insurmountable heights and unimaginable beauty.

This was about a love that runs as deep as it does wide. Like drilling our well, and not stopping when we first hit water, but holding onto hope and digging deeper, breaking through to an artesian well that gave abundant water. Through this devastating illness, we had tapped into the well of love itself, the kind that is abundantly supplied from only one source.

> There's a love that's divine
> And it's yours and it's mine
> It shines like the sun.
> At the end of the day
> We should give thanks and pray
> To the One.
> ~Van Morrison, *Have I told You Lately That I Love You?*

§

One simple man, one deadly disease, thousands of lives touched.

The math doesn't make sense. At least not until you put it in the perspective of a small rock.

Troy was the rock tossed into the pool. The disease was the first ripple that encompassed him.

The next circle is the family, a part of the ripple effect of anything that touches Troy.

The next circle is friends, then the church, then the community, and ultimately the world as the circles get bigger and bigger. Troy would be the first to tell you that he was just an ordinary man — with an extraordinary disease. But combined with his commitment to life, to love, and to leaving a legacy for his family, he showed us all what one man's life can do.

15
SO FEW WORDS...SO MUCH SAID

Do not go where the path may lead;
go instead where there is no path and leave a trail.
~Ralph Waldo Emerson

Now, nearly four years after Troy's diagnosis, I found myself leading a kind woman in a blue suit into our bedroom. The chosen cameraman was setting up a large microphone above the bed. A smaller one was given to me to attach to my blouse. The woman was Nancy Francis, the news anchor from Channel 8. There were three other reporters lined up across the foot of the bed, notepads in hand. Together they represented the four major television networks in Portland.

Troy's eyes were so alert, so alive. He was ready for this! I was not so sure I was. But I didn't have a choice — I was his mouthpiece to the outside world.

I noticed as I reached over to take Troy's hand that my hands were cold and clammy. He noticed it, too, and gave me a smile of encouragement. He was so calm! How did he do it?

Thankfully, Josh brought me a glass of water as things were about to get started. I had learned the hard way what nervousness can do to your mouth when you try to speak in front of an audience. I had been asked to speak about Troy's illness for a group of high school students at West Linn, Troy's old high school. I no sooner got started then my mouth got so dry, I felt like I had been licking a pool table!

"Are we ready?" the cameraman asked the group. Around the crowded room heads nodded in reply.

"Okay everyone, here we go."

§

After the Oregonian published our story, we were growing more used to the idea of living in a fishbowl. In addition to the international interviews, our local Newberg paper did a big story. But things took on a whole new dimension the day Troy agreed to be a plaintiff in a lawsuit challenging the state of Oregon's Measure 16, legalizing physician-assisted suicide.

Early in March of 1998, the Physicians for Compassionate care, which included one of Troy's team of doctors, Dr. Miles Edwards, contacted us, asking Troy if he would consider being a plaintiff in the lawsuit.

A similar lawsuit had been thrown out by the 9th Circuit Court of Appeals on the grounds that the law did not directly affect the plaintiff(s) in the case, and they were therefore not qualified to sue. In other words, all the doctors, attorneys, and various other professionals who had joined in the first lawsuit opposing Ballot Measure 16 were not qualified because none of them were terminally ill.

So the next step was to find someone who was terminally ill to agree to be the plaintiff.

A man named Peter Begin agreed to do it. They had the second lawsuit already in process when the proposed plaintiff died. The case was to be heard in the US District court in Eugene, Oregon on April 14, 1998 in front of Judge Michael Hogan.

Now with less than six weeks until the scheduled hearing, Troy was asked if he would consider being the new plaintiff. Dr. Edwards asked us to think about it, and shortly after we were contacted by the team of attorneys.

In a conference call with the attorneys, they explained the basis for the lawsuit and what Troy's role would be. I would act as power of attorney for Troy in signing documents, be his voice for depositions, and represent him at the hearings. There would be no financial costs to us. They told us to take a couple days to think about it, even though time was running short.

I wasn't so sure about all of this. My concern was for Troy's extremely fragile health, not to mention the thought of taking on one more thing. It was hard to imagine how we could add another thing to our overflowing plate.

But my husband was looking at the big picture. He typed out on his computer: "For evil to prevail is for good men to do nothing."

He agreed to do the lawsuit.

§

In a matter of days, the Oregonian picked up the story about Troy and the lawsuit. Once that hit the newspaper, the phone again started ringing off the hook.

Every television station in town called for an interview. We decided the best way to handle it for Troy's sake was to invite them to come all at once. With the approval of the attorneys, we set it up for 9:30 a.m. Friday morning, April 3.

Besides the local television networks, we had calls from all over the country! TV stations, magazines, radio, and newspapers were all following the story. I couldn't believe it. I agreed to a couple of interviews at first. One was the national Catholic Newspaper from Florida called "Our Sunday

Visitor." Another was a radio spot for Family News and Focus out of Colorado Springs.

I was becoming so overwhelmed, I had to start saying no, even when USA Today called.

A number of newspapers around the country picked it up from the Associated Press and ran the story. I have no idea how many. But we received phone calls of support from as far away as Maryland and British Columbia.

It still amazes me when I think about how calm Troy was that day when the television crews swarmed into our house. It had just been a few weeks before when Troy had asked me a startling question.

"Have I made it...as a husband?" he had spelled out as we shared an especially intimate moment, struggling for the right words. I was surprised by the question.

"Of course Hon," I replied. "Of course you have."

What he needed to know was that he had fulfilled his role as a husband and not disappointed me with the physical limitations he had. Men rely so much on their physical body to protect, love, and care for their wife, and too often strength is defined by physical attributes.

I told him that he had become the strongest man I knew. His love and encouragement went beyond anything I had ever experienced.

And here he was now, with all the activity going on around us in this crowded bedroom, and he was giving me a smile that felt like there was no one else in the room but us...

§

At 5:00 that evening the family piled onto our bed, all eyes focused eagerly on the television set we had wheeled into the bedroom for the occasion. We set up VCRs on two other TVs so we could record the other stations at the same time.

The camera zoomed in on the news reporter, papers in hand, dressed in a dark suit and red tie.

"Our top story tonight, Troy is 36 years old and suffering from Lou Gehrig's disease. We take you to the home of Troy Thompson where a dramatic scene unfolds.

"Paralyzed by a disease that will eventually take his life, this man, with his wife by his side voicing his views, is ready to take on the legal fight *against* doctor-assisted suicide.

"Some might think the man you are about to meet would want to take advantage of the assisted suicide law.

"Instead, Troy Thompson has agreed to serve as the plaintiff in a lawsuit to stop Oregon's highly controversial physician-assisted suicide law.

"Tonight as he struggles to live, Troy is trying to make sure others don't die prematurely."

The story was being aired across all four of the major networks as the lead story in the evening news. Some of the stations ran it again on the 6:00 news, and again at 11:00. Each one was a slightly different version, telling the story using different things I had said and different photographs they had taken from our collection of when Troy was healthy.

"Troy Thompson's life changed dramatically three and a half years ago when he was diagnosed with ALS, better known as Lou Gehrig's disease. The deterioration is unmistakable, irreversible, and places a premium on life," said another reporter. "Now his wife makes careful efforts to understand her husband, and speak for him. Using a system of eye blinks and a chart of letters, Troy explains why he wants to fight Oregon's assisted suicide law."

The camera moves from the newsroom to our bedroom. "It's hard for Troy not to feel like a burden to us," I am saying. "He is afraid that with this new law, pressure may be put on people who dread being a burden, physically and financially, to end their lives sooner. Our experience has been extraordinary. Living day to day, you realize what your priorities are. What is important. To have missed this experience...well...there have been very, very hard things. And on the other hand, there have been some profound things."

On another station, I was shown saying, "He said the pressure and the waiting, not knowing when you're going to die, has been very hard. But he would have missed so much. We value life...every day of life."

The camera moves to a shot of Victoria, sitting on the bed next to Troy in her red dress.

The reporter continues, "Like being with Victoria, his four-year-old daughter. She doesn't remember the days when her Daddy could hold her, but he does. He felt great sadness when he heard about the two Oregonians who recently took their lives under the new law."

A cheer went up from our bedroom when all four stations ran his most important quote.

"I think Troy said it best," I told the reporters, "When he said, 'God doesn't make mistakes, we do. God is the author and finisher of our life.'"

Seeing myself sitting on that familiar stool next to the bed, being my husband's voice, I was struck by the heartbreaking whirlwind that had taken place in our lives in such a short time...

§

As seems to typically happen with court cases, the date for the hearing was postponed to May 8th, and then again to July 14th, a four-month delay. The attorneys were optimistic that if Judge Hogan ruled in our favor, there would be a preliminary injunction against Measure 16. They anticipated the case to "heat up quickly" and go before the U.S. Court of Appeals for the 9th Circuit and possibly the U.S. Supreme court within a few months.

Meanwhile, the clock was still running for Troy. I would have given anything to stop that clock, to make time stand still until a cure was found for ALS. We continued to hold onto hope, but his health was visibly deteriorating. For the past couple of months he had been having breathing episodes where his breathing would stop, as if he was holding his breath.

Panic filled his eyes, and then after five to six seconds he would wince in pain as his body involuntarily exhaled. He would take two to three larger, quick breaths and his breathing would return to normal.

When Dr. Edwards came to see Troy in March, he again reiterated that "it was truly amazing that he has survived this long." The breathing spells were increasing. He explained that the muscles in his lungs were growing weaker, and involuntarily stopping for a few seconds.

We tried different oxygen masks and external ways to get him additional oxygen, short of a ventilator. But none of them were comfortable for him. He just couldn't tolerate anything covering his face or mouth.

The only thing that was tolerable, but not much help, was these nose "plugs" that delivered oxygen through a tube hooked up to an oxygen tank. It's the kind you see people using occasionally out in public where they are carrying or sometimes wheeling a portable tank with them.

What seemed to help the most was increasing his morphine. It allowed his muscles to relax instead of panic during these spells so he could get his breathing started again.

§

One evening Troy was having more difficulty than normal with the breathing spells. Josh had already gone home, and Victoria was in bed. I remember the night well. It was

May 17th, and it was still light outside, even though it was around eight o'clock.

During one of the breathing spells, five or six seconds went by and Troy didn't start breathing again. Several more seconds went by and still nothing. His eyes showed the same terror that I was feeling. His skin was rapidly turning an alarming purple color.

In a panic, I fumbled with his feeding tube, trying to get more morphine in using the little eyedropper and spilling half the bottle on the dresser. Still, he wasn't breathing.

Using the remote to turn on the speakerphone, I used speed dial to call Josh. Thank God Josh was home and answered after two rings.

"Josh! You've got to get over here fast. Troy's not breathing!" I screamed at the phone from across the room.

I remembered the oxygen tank that we had stuck in a corner of the den. It wasn't one of the small, portable kinds. I ran to the den and dragged that heavy steel tank with both hands across the wood floor and into the bedroom. The whole time I was screaming to Troy to hold on.

"You're not going to die!" I yelled to him as I fumbled with all the tubing and nozzles, trying desperately to remember how to set up the tank. His face was now totally purple, and I could see that he was losing consciousness.

Just as I was getting the oxygen going through the tubing, he miraculously started to breathe again. His breathing was labored, but his color was starting to return. I looked into his eyes and could see that he had regained consciousness and knew what was going on. He was back! My husband, my soul mate...was alive!!!

Just then, we heard sirens coming up the hill. I looked out the large bedroom window and could see several vehicles including ambulances and a fire truck coming up the hill towards our neighborhood, red lights flashing, sirens blaring.

Troy's eyes grew wide again with dismay. I knew he didn't like the whole ambulance thing. Apparently Josh had called them.

Josh flew in the door just ahead of the paramedics. Troy's color had returned to normal. The whole episode had left him weak and he was having difficulty breathing normally, but the crisis was over.

Josh opened the front door for the paramedics, and as was typical, at least eight men swept into the bedroom. Josh started giving details to one of them who was taking notes, while another came to the bedside to see what he could do.

Everything they would have been able to do, using the oxygen and narcotics, had already been done.

I apologized for their trouble, but as usual, they were very kind and understanding.

"That's what we're here for," said the guy who seemed to be in charge. "Don't ever hesitate to call us...anytime."

Another guy asked as he was leaving if we were the people he had seen on TV.

One of the truly amazing things through this whole incident was Victoria. She never woke up! Her bedroom is right below ours, and with that many men stomping into our bedroom, not to mention the sirens, it was unbelievable that she slept through it all.

We found out later that Dana, one of her little friends on our street, had heard the sirens and had been frightened to tears. Yet Victoria was protected from the trauma and never heard a thing...

§

How do I describe what it was like, living under the shadow of death? So many times, I almost lost him. And then we would be given the gift of one more day, one more week, one more month.

The toll physically and emotionally was enormous. For the most part, my health stood the test, but I knew there would be a price to pay. You can't put your body through that level of strain and stress for four years and not pay a price down the road. I knew it would come.

One of the hardest struggles was not being able to ever be fully rested. I was just trying to put one foot in front of the other. To drag myself out of bed each day, wishing I could sleep another few hours — twenty-four would be good. I fell into bed at night, bone weary, with that constant anxiety that I probably wouldn't get to sleep without interruption.

No one else lived with it physically, seven days a week, like I did. Josh could go home at night and on the weekends (most of the time). Troy's Mom would come on the weekends and leave on Sunday, drained, to go back to her own home. Her own bed. Her freedom to watch a TV show or take a bath.

How I longed to spend an evening reading a book or watching a movie without interruptions every fifteen minutes. Or maybe go out to dinner once in awhile. In four years, I had maybe been out to dinner three or four times. I never left the house after I got home from work. I forgot what it was like to even drive a car after dark.

But if I ever started feeling sorry for myself, all I had to do was look at my husband.

He could never get *out* of bed. Going out to dinner? What he would have given to taste just one meal...To drive his sports car...To stand under a hot shower and feel the water pouring over his body...To pick up his little girl and toss her in the air...To wrap his arms around his wife. If even just for a day...

The toughest challenge I faced while continuing to work full time throughout these four years wasn't getting up and going to work each day. That was actually a break in which I had time to myself on the drive to work. Being at work was a needed distraction.

The true challenge was watching other people living normal lives. Not just seeing couples with their arms around each other, although that did cause a twinge in my heart.

It was hearing people complain that the whole day was ruined because the copy machine wasn't working.

Or grumble that their spouse had left their clothes on the bathroom floor.

Or say they were getting bored with their marriage or they weren't getting along, and maybe it was time to make a change.

It was heartbreaking to watch couples throw away their marriage when they had a choice. Short of death, there is always hope.

§

The next day I had only been at work for an hour when Troy had Josh call and ask me to come home. He rarely did that, but it had been such a frightening experience the night before. He needed to see me, to just be together. I badly needed to be with him, too, afraid of not being there with him if this were to happen again. I cancelled all appointments and went home.

16
A DEER IN THE GARDEN

"Hold everything in your hands lightly,
otherwise it hurts when God pries your fingers open."
~Corrie ten Boom

A season of changes had arrived again. They seemed to blow through in gusts. This time it was the caregivers — again. Diane told us that she was going to have to cut way back on her hours in order to take care of her new grandchild.

Janice, another night nurse, was starting summer school so we were back to looking for replacements. Patti, our hospice volunteer, was moving to Portland and would no longer be able to come on Wednesdays.

To top it off, our insurance money had just run out. For the rest of the year, we would be using what was left of our savings. We had already sold the rental house to make ends meet last year, and this time we put the beach house up for sale.

Three weeks after our latest brush with death was Victoria's fifth birthday. Another goal reached, another landmark. It looked as if Troy was going to make it to see her start kindergarten after all.

While Bert, Victoria's godfather, worked up a sweat trying to assemble the basketball hoop they had given her for her birthday, Josh and I took turns taking care of Troy.

We had the party in the living room this time. Troy wasn't up to having visitors lately. On top of the breathing difficulties, he had developed an eye infection that was so severe his whole eye was swollen shut.

With the one eye unable to open, Troy was too weak to keep the other one open. And with his eye-blinks our main source of communication these days, it was extremely frustrating. We struggled to figure out what he needed to say.

Finally, we found a way for him to tell us "yes" or "no" by a barely perceptible movement of his leg. Even then, he couldn't always do that when he was tired.

Even when Troy's dad came from Arizona for Father's Day, he hardly ever opened his eyes. Without being able to look into his eyes, without his smile, I was missing him desperately. It was almost as if he was already gone. He slept most of the time as his body tried to fight off the infection.

Then, after a couple of weeks, he opened his eyes. I was so thrilled! His eye still looked terrible, but he managed to open it for short periods.

On June 24th, Josh's dad had a heart attack and Josh had to leave that night for Arizona. Even through these tough few weeks, the scales kept re-balancing through the love of others.

Troy's dad and Uncle Mose (short for Maurice), built a playhouse for Victoria. My neighbor mowed the fields for me.

Connie and Steve became good friends after we moved to Newberg. Their daughter, Monica, was Victoria's best friend and playmate from pre-school. They were so helpful with Victoria through these four years. Without them, Victoria would have missed so much. She liked to call Steve "daddy," even though she would sometimes get a sideways look of disapproval from Monica.

Connie would take Victoria to swim classes and gymnastics, and take the girls to the park or horseback riding on Monica's pony. I cannot say enough about what a relief it was for Troy and I to have help with our daughter. Not just babysitting, but knowing that she was able to carry on normal activities. It was an invaluable gift to us for her to have those opportunities when our hands were tied. At times, I could not help but feel cheated. There was so much I longed to do with Troy. Or even just by myself.

On the 4th of July, Monica's family took Victoria to the St. Paul rodeo and fireworks show. I wanted so much to go with them, to watch the excitement in my little girl's eyes when she saw her first rodeo, and to sit on the grass and hold her in my lap under a blanket while we watched the fireworks.

Instead, I sat on the deck by myself, and watched as fireworks were going off across the valley. I could see off in the distance the display going on at the rodeo.

It was a perfect summer night, still warm at 10:00 p.m. I sat in the dark, the house lights blazing behind me.

I could see Troy through the bedroom window where the light was still on. He wasn't asleep, but I didn't feel like going inside to sit with him and have to take care of all the things he would ask for. I just wanted to sit here alone in the dark and feel the warm night air.

How could I have known that one week later he would be gone?

§

After several minutes, I felt guilty for leaving him alone. I pulled myself away from the view of the city lights and the popping fireworks, and went inside. When I went inside to check on him, and spend the last part of the holiday with him, he had gone to sleep. I sat down on the stool beside the bed as loneliness set in like a cold, damp fog.

I was stuck in a crevasse, not able to get to the top on either side. On one side were life's normal activities — work, play.

On the other side was my husband. Even when I tried to be with Troy, lately it was as if he was not really there. Either asleep, or unable to communicate, I was losing the one part of his body the disease hadn't taken away…his mind.

Many times, I have wondered what it must be like for the families of Alzheimer victims. I would come to the conclusion that I would rather have Troy paralyzed with his mind intact, than unable to recognize me.

One of the hardest things to reconcile was how young Troy was. So many diseases such as Alzheimer's strike the elderly. Terrible as it is, usually they are reaching the end of their lives already. We are all going to die sometime. Having to live without loved ones is a normal part of life.

And the "losses" start right from birth. We watch our children grow and within weeks of being born, they are no longer a "newborn.' They change from an infant to a toddler in a short period of time, and then to pre-school kids. *They will never be babies again.* It is gone forever.

What they change into by junior high does not even closely resemble what they were a few short years before! We lose our babies, our hair, our youth, our hearing, and our elasticity. Without realizing it, we are grieving losses all through our lives.

I would try to tell myself that it just came sooner for Troy — that I would have eventually had to give up his ability to carry me up the stairs to our bedroom, or working in the garden side by side until we were covered in sweat and dirt.

But the losses came so fast, so cruelly. I couldn't look at him lying there, sleeping, knowing the end was near, and feel the satisfaction of having lived a long life together. I couldn't rest in the comfort of knowing that if he died first, I would be following him soon. At times, I would grow envious of his mother, because she was older and the odds were she would get to see Troy again, after he was gone, a lot sooner than I would.

God, I'm older than Troy! I shouldn't have to be the one left alone. I shouldn't have to be a single parent…again. *It's not supposed to be this way!*

§

The next Friday night, a week after the 4th of July, I had another of those rare moments alone. Victoria had gone to spend the night with Michelle at her home in Salem where she lived with her mom and step dad. It was the first time Victoria had gotten to do this, and she was so excited when she hugged me good-bye.

I sat down to eat my dinner of leftovers, and read the paper. Josh had just left, relieved that the weekend was here. He was looking forward to going fishing on Saturday.

The phone rang. It was Victoria's pediatrician.

"How is Troy's eye doing?" she asked. She had already sent a doctor friend of hers to the house to look at it.

"It's not a lot better," I told her. "And what are you doing calling at 6:30 on a Friday night? Shouldn't you have gone home by now?"

"Yes, yes," she replied in her distinctive German accent. "I just wanted to make sure he was doing okay before the weekend."

I thanked her for her concern, and she promised to have another doctor get in touch with me on Monday to come and check on him.

I started again to read the paper, and noticed that the sounds coming over the monitor from Troy's room were unusual. The sounds were so soft they were barely audible.

But something was not right. In that moment I realized that he was in trouble. I jumped up from the table and rushed to the bedroom. I found Troy in a state of distress, his breathing shallow and fast. He was clearly not getting enough air, and was growing weaker by the second. I paged Josh, who hadn't even made it home yet from the errands he was running for me.

When Josh arrived, Troy's condition had not changed. Not sure what was going to happen, I called Troy's Mom and Pastor Keith to come over.

Things were not improving. We used the oxygen tank, increased his morphine, everything we could think of. But nothing was helping. Grasping at straws, I called Ellen, who had been helping work on Troy with alternative health care methods. She came right over, but there wasn't a lot that could be done for Troy except to pray. And hope.

Close to midnight, Keith and Ellen went home. Troy's condition was not changing. He seemed fairly peaceful; although I now know he was only semi-conscious. His coloring looked good, but Josh knew that was only because of the oxygen we were giving him.

Josh realized when he arrived that night what was happening: respiratory failure.

He and Dr. Johnston had been in agreement that Troy had been in a downward spiral since these respiratory episodes had started a few months ago, and that Troy had reached the outer limits of his ability to function. But Troy and I had chosen not to give up hope. Not until his last breath.

I pleaded with Troy not to stop breathing, to keep fighting.

"Don't give up!" I begged him.

I couldn't possibly imagine that he would die now. Not two days before the trial! *What was God thinking?!*

But his breathing continued in those short, weak breaths, as he lay with his eyes closed and no responses to our coaxing. Troy's mom and I cried and wailed as we took turns holding Troy's hand and caressing his face.

Mom implored Josh to do something! Couldn't he do *something*? Anything?

Slowly the breathing grew fainter until it stopped… And Troy was gone.

§

At 3:30 a.m. on Saturday morning, July 11, 1998, Troy took his final breath. I wandered around the house in shock. In a daze, I went from the bedroom to the living room, and back to the bedroom.

Troy lay there with his eyes closed, looking like he always did when he slept. I sat by his side and held his hand, kissing his face.

I just couldn't believe this body had no life in it. After all the hundreds of hours and days and weeks that I had cared for this body, it couldn't possibly be over. There must still be *something* I could do for him.

I wandered out onto the deck. It was 5:30 in the morning and the sun was just starting to come up.

Looking over the rail into the yard below I was startled to see a deer standing there, not twenty feet from me. It was a huge buck with a full rack of antlers.

He looked up at me, his gaze unflinching. We stood there and looked at each other for what seemed like several minutes. Then he peacefully, majestically walked down the hill and across the drive. He stopped at the rose garden for a minute and then slowly moved on, out of sight.

I didn't quite know what to make of it. We have had deer in our yard before, but the instant they spot you or catch your scent, they bound off into the woods. And I had never seen one so big, with that many antlers.

Mike Wiltshire, one of my sales agents, had a similar experience. He lived in Newberg also, on the next "mountain" over. That same morning he had noticed a family of deer come into his back yard. He, too, has a couple of acres. In fact, Troy had done the landscape design for Mike's new house. It was the last one Troy did besides our own.

Mike had seen deer in his yard before, too, but what was unusual about this day was that they didn't leave once the sun came out and exposed their resting place. Mike was amazed when this family of deer stayed the whole day in his back yard.

It was not until he found out that Troy had died that morning, and that I had a similar experience, that he realized the significance. We both knew that there was a message in the undaunted peacefulness the deer had experienced.

§

We gathered the family together that morning at the house. Keith came back, and Bert came over. I will forever be thankful that Victoria was spared that night. It was the only night she has ever spent at Michelle's house, and I found it very comforting that they were together that night. I asked that the girls be brought home after the coroners had come and gone.

Of all the things we went through, from the day we got the diagnosis, through all the crises, nothing was as horrible for me as this final hour when the coroners came and took Troy away.

I wasn't prepared for this.

I had never mentally imagined this moment ahead of time. When they wheeled Troy's body out of our bedroom and paused in the foyer to open the double front doors, I experienced the most anguished, helpless feeling imaginable.

I was still in a state of shock and disbelief from his breathing having stopped just hours before. Somehow it seemed like he might just start breathing again. We had been at the edge of death so many times, and made it back again.

To see these strangers taking away my husband was more than I could bear. I wanted to stop them, to keep him here longer — to keep taking care of him.

I screamed in anguish as Bert held me. Deep, racking sobs like I had never experienced before shook my whole being.

§

If you have experienced the death of a loved one, you know the odd dream-like state that takes over for the next several days as you plan the funeral.

It becomes a busy time of phone calls, visitors, decisions, and plans. Planning a funeral in some ways is like planning a wedding. There is the church, music, ushers, flowers, the press release, and all the people to "invite." The tasks are a welcome diversion to holding back the grief. And Troy had wanted a full-on funeral, complete with pallbearers whom he had selected ahead of time.

One of the tasks I had to do was to call the attorneys on Sunday, the day before the trial, and tell them that the plaintiff had just died.

I know that God sees a bigger picture than we do, but still, the timing of Troy's death was so baffling. The attorneys were wonderfully supportive, and assured me that even though Troy wouldn't be there on Monday, his life and the way he lived it had already done a great deal for getting his message out on the sanctity of life.

I agonized over whether to make the trip to Eugene on Monday for the trial, but decided I needed to be at home with the family. It would still go on even without Troy as the attorneys moved for a class action suit that would allow several plaintiffs to join the suit, for the obvious reasons of what had just happened to Troy.

Hundreds of people attended the funeral, including his hospice team, doctors, and media people. The newspapers had carried the story with headlines that read "Suicide Plaintiff Dies Before Hearing." Pastor Ron Mehl did an awesome job, as did Keith Reetz, Bert Waugh, Ted Nelson, and Shad Williams who all spoke. And even Troy "spoke."

Just two days before the funeral I had been on Troy's computer looking for a document. My breath caught in my throat when I ran across a letter he had written called **"Good-Bye for Now"**:

> "If you are reading this, it is because I'm no longer with you, but home with our Lord. I have been so blessed by all of you and want to **thank you** all very much. You all are the second greatest gift God has given me. Of course, second only to the gift of salvation through his son, Jesus Christ. I have been very fortunate to have such a wonderful wife and friend, Marilyn."

Somehow I don't think the letter was finished. But that would be typical of Troy. He wasn't always the best at finishing projects. He always had good intentions, but ...

Following the large funeral at the church, we had a small gathering of family and close friends at the gravesite. As the last few friends laid flowers on the casket and walked back to their cars, I noticed Ryan off to the side. He was struggling. Not only with the emotional day we had just been through, but with the larger question of why?

Ryan was angry. Angry with God. How could a God who is supposed to be a loving father allow this to happen? If he is omnipotent, why didn't he stop this?! Why is it that it always seems like the really good people in life end up with the most suffering? Maybe there really isn't a God at all.

Ryan and Troy had been especially close. When Ryan and Summer started dating, and later became great friends, Troy was excited to have another male around. They had great times watching movies together (the sci-fi kind that Summer and I don't like).

I still laugh when I think of the trip to our beach house and the crabbing expedition. Watching Ryan learn how to clean his first crabs was "Saturday Night Live" material for sure.

Ryan was away at college in California during the time of Troy's illness. He kept in touch by writing letters, and visited whenever he came home.

Troy continued to try to encourage him in his faith. But with the heartbreaking progression of the disease and then Troy's death, Ryan was at a crossroads. It's a place that a lot of people come to in their lives, but witnessing such a personal tragedy and loss was a catalyst.

Ryan, you need to know something. And as I type, I can sense Troy looking over my shoulder. You are very special to Troy. He thought of you almost like a younger brother. He loves you and your family so much, and would have done anything for you. He would have given his life for you, Ryan. I know him. He would go through the whole thing again if he thought it would have meant that he would see you again one day in heaven. And he's not the only one who feels this way. Someone else already gave his life for you, two thousand years ago. Just for you.

Troy's life is only a tragedy if it causes someone to lose their faith. We can't understand God's ways. It's okay to ask why; I certainly do. And occasionally God, in his great compassion, answers that question, giving us a little glimpse into how our lives fit in to the bigger plan. We don't see the big picture, but he does. Thankfully, I have been given at least a small glimpse into several peoples' lives that were changed by Troy's journey. This life we know now is only a moment in time compared to eternity.

And Ryan, Troy has a *lot* more movies he wants to watch with you one day.

§

As was true in his life, in his death Troy impacted and changed lives. His funeral service had life-changing impact on several people. But my favorite was Josh…

Before he came to work for us, Josh had been struggling with direction for his life, with relationships, with his faith.

It was at Troy's funeral that Josh made the decision to give his life over to Jesus Christ.

And it was at Troy's funeral that Josh met the woman he would marry a year later, on our deck, with a 16x24" picture of Troy propped on a chair as his best man.

Josh had lost not only a job, but also his best friend. He had no idea what he was going to do for work, but most of all what he was supposed to do emotionally.

His relationship with Troy was a rare and priceless gift. Sometimes Troy was like a father to him, sometimes like a brother. Like me, Josh could tell what Troy was thinking before he even tried to communicate it.

Spending that much time being someone else's hands, feet, mouth, and protector caused a phenomenon that later was difficult for Josh to put into words. It was as if part of him became Troy. And in the process, Josh lost sight of who he was without Troy.

It would take several months before Josh understood what was happening, but just like me, he needed to truly grasp that it wasn't Troy who was his hero and best friend. It was actually Jesus, living through Troy's life, that Josh had grown to love and depend on.

Troy was always the first to remind me of that when, through tears, I would say things like, "I don't know how I'm going to go on without you."

He would assure me that I was going to be okay, that he wasn't my source of strength. "Don't forget, I'm not perfect. I make mistakes, and let you down sometimes. But God never will."

17
NEVER, EVER, GIVE UP

"Life is a gift. Living it is a choice."
~Author Unknown

We may not get to choose our life, when and where we are born, or who our parents are. If you really think about it, as pastor Ron would say, life is totally out of control—at least out of our control.

When you wake up in the morning, you have no idea what that day may bring. What we do have control over, though, is the choice to live life. First, to live life every day, to its fullest. And second, to live every day of our lives to the last.

"All the days ordained for me were written in your book before one of them came to be" (Psalms 139:16).

This second point is what became the center of the extremely controversial issue in the state of Oregon, and really, around the world.

In 1994, when Oregon passed the law allowing physician-assisted suicide, the voters in Oregon were persuaded with convincing arguments that stated doctors should be allowed to assist the dying when they had a terminal illness, and no longer wanted to go on living. They were told this was the compassionate thing to do. The law defines a terminal illness as being diagnosed by a doctor and having less than six months to live. The law allows for doctors to prescribe lethal drugs to someone who is terminally ill and of a sound mind.

The supporters of the bill called it "The Death with Dignity Act." And it was argued that it gives the control back to the individual—the control over when to die.

That sounds good, doesn't it?

Being compassionate with the terminally ill?

Of course! "Dying with dignity?" Certainly. We would all like that. Having control over the day of our death?

For that matter, how about control over our whole life?

This whole issue starts to play into the arena that is core to our very being. Are we, or *should* we be, in control of life and death?

To Oregonians, at least on the surface, it sounded simple. Compassionate, dignified. Taking control of our death. But it is the tip of the iceberg to a much larger issue.

One of the obvious problems is that it is not exactly taking control of our death. What the law did was make it legal for someone else to take control of our death—doctors.

In a perfect world, maybe. With 100% accurate medical diagnosis, and a perfect legal system to protect the patient from the unscrupulous. It would also need to be a world without greed, where family members and insurance companies did not influence decisions based on financial circumstances. But if it were a perfect world, there would not be any disease or suffering.

In the state of Oregon, a group called Physicians for Compassionate Care has been active in promoting compassionate care of the dying, rather than assisting them to die prematurely. They have as their pledge:

We will treat the sick according to our best ability and
judgement,
always striving to do no harm.
We will give comfort care until natural death.
We will support our patients' wishes not to prolong
the dying process with futile care.
We will never give a deadly drug to anyone even if
asked,
nor will we suggest suicide.
Whatever we see or hear in the course of medical
practice,
we will keep private and confidential.
With integrity, we will always affirm and guard these
ethical principles
recognizing that every human life is inherently
valuable.

The message is clear. We should be focusing on ways to
help people live out their last days. Not cut them short…by
their will or against it.

Troy's life was a stellar example of the flawed thinking
that physician assisted suicide represents.

If he had been tempted by the availability of assistance
from his doctor in ending his life, and had decided to give up
when things started getting really tough, his life could have
been cut short by *two and a half years*.

Troy was given less than six months to live in
December of 1995, which made him eligible to go on hospice.

Think of it.

Troy was on hospice for two and a half years! I think he
was one of the longest running patients they ever had.

In studying this issue, one of the primary reasons
people request the narcotics from their physician that will end
their lives is for the security of knowing that they will have

that option if things get too difficult. It's about fear of the future and the inevitable suffering they have ahead of them.

Troy and I can empathize with that fear and suffering in a very real and personal way. But we can also testify to the amazing experiences, relationships, and impact of one's life that someone who considers suicide risks missing.

A fellow ALS widow, Kathy, shared with me that during her husband's battle with Lou Gehrig's, she had been in favor of Ballot Measure 16 and assisted suicide. But after her experience of going through her husband's final days and his death, her opinions changed.

"I wouldn't have wanted to miss those last three weeks for anything in the world," Kathy told me. "You just can't imagine it until you've been through it."

Who could have predicted that Troy would outlive the doctor's prognosis by over two years? His doctors were very competent, and we believe they gave their best medical prognosis.

If we really stop and think about it, when has life ever gone the way we thought it would?

I know mine sure hasn't! I would not have ever predicted that both my parents would have died before I would reach the age of 40. I would never in my wildest dreams have imagined that my knight in shining armor would be gone six years after we were married.

All of us can look back and see the unexpected twists and turns of life. It is looking forward that we are not equipped to do. That is the job of someone far more capable than we mortals are.

We marvel at what we would have missed had Troy taken advantage of assisted suicide when he was eligible. In those last two years of his life, Troy had a profound influence on more lives, including mine, than he had in his entire thirty-four years prior.

God has much bigger plans than we have. "He who is able to do immeasurably more than we ask or imagine, according to his power that is at work within us" (Ephesians 3:20).

Was it easy? Of course not. Was it dignified? Not most of the time. Some of the things that we had to do in caring for Troy go way beyond what any of us want to even think about.

But Troy's message was loud and clear: When things get tough in life, you don't quit.

Troy especially had a heart for young people. Yes, Paul Linnman was right when he said this world needs role models. Troy lived his life to send the message that when things start getting really tough, do not quit. Drugs, guns, or suicide is not the answer.

And the choices we make today, big and small, will have an effect not only on those around us today, but on future generations as well.

Every decision you make is writing history. The way we live our life is writing the legacy we will leave.

18
A ROSE IN FULL BLOOM

"When a blossom's fragrance is at its height,
the rose in full bloom takes a glorious place in the garden."
~Anonymous

If there is one thing that rises to the top for me as the most significant life-lesson of this journey, it is the potential two people have in a marriage relationship to experience a love like none other. Too many people throw away that opportunity.

I know now that it is not the love that comes during courtship, or what we experience at the altar. It is so much deeper than that. It is the rich love that comes by fire.

I'm not talking about the fire of passion. It's the fire that comes from going through the trials of life — the fire of testing where the gold is separated from the dross and we are left purer, more brilliant, than before.

Every marriage is going to twist and turn through tough times, whether with each other or from outside circumstances.

Troy and I would not have willingly volunteered for Lou Gehrig's disease. I would never wish it on anyone in a million years.

But the fact is, that was our course and by staying on it rather than looking at alternatives, such as divorce, our love grew into a deeper bond and increased our commitment to each other.

Don't walk away from the challenges in your marriage.

Don't try to figure out a way around them. It is by walking straight through that you find the joy waiting on the other side for you.

When Troy and I married, each for the second time, we both felt like we had been given a second chance. A chance to do things right this time, each having experienced the pain and sorrow of failed marriages and broken children. Our hope and prayer was that our marriage would be one that would maybe be a guiding light to others. Who knows? Maybe someday we would even counsel other couples or lead a workshop on marriage.

But instead we were struggling. It's not easy blending families together. As a matter of fact, at times it was pure hell. Especially with teenage daughters who wanted nothing to do with this intrusion in their lives that was taking their mother's time and attention away from them.

We sought the counsel of Pastor Keith to try to help with the distance that was starting to grow between us as we closed ourselves off from the stress and from each other.

Our prayer for our marriage was answered — but in a most unexpected way. Our life was not turning out to be the Cinderella love story we had hoped for.

Instead, we were faced with the most difficult challenge either of us could imagine. A tragic death sentence like Lou Gehrig's disease changes everything. Suddenly all our other problems seemed small.

We would gladly have re-wound the tape and taken back our "old issues."

You know the ones. The husband who spends too much time watching TV (his hideout from stress) instead of spending the time with his wife.

Or the differences of opinion on how to deal with the rebellious teenager or the attention seeking five-year-old.

Or the disagreements over finances.

The list goes on, as it does in all marriages. But all of a sudden these problems seemed so small, so insignificant.

We were getting a second chance at marriage all right. In a culture where words are cheap and selfishness reigns, we were suddenly thrown into a situation that demanded sacrifice, unwavering commitment, and unconditional love.

But that's what a marriage is supposed to be all about in the first place.

Real love, the deep love, comes with a price. True love may be called priceless. Or there is the old saying that the best things in life are free.

I disagree. They aren't free. But they are worth the price.

§

Troy loved roses. Of all the flowers in the garden, the rose was his favorite. For a wedding present, he gave me a rose garden of pale pink, Old English roses.

One of the many things I loved about Troy was that he was a true, unabashed romantic. He was always giving me roses. His trademark was to give me a dozen red roses with one white one in the center, symbolic of a God-centered relationship.

Troy loved giving gifts and surprises.

One Valentine's Day a dozen pink roses arrived. I admit, I was expecting the roses, but was surprised by the pink. But that wasn't the surprise. A few hours later another dozen roses arrived! Red, of course, with one white…

Even after he could no longer order the flowers or deliver them in person, he had Josh or his mom order them.

On our sixth anniversary, Mom was ordering flowers from the usual florist when she learned a heart-warming story of how Troy's illness had impacted another marriage.

The owner of the shop recognized Troy's name on the order, and shared with Mom her story...

She had lost her husband to a sudden death a year before. Since then, she had met a wonderful man, Frank, and they planned to be married. Shortly after their engagement, he became ill.

After weeks of testing, Frank was diagnosed with the same dreaded disease...ALS. They decided to call the wedding off.

A few weeks later, the article in the Oregonian came out about us. They were so inspired by our courage and strength that they made the decision to "risk it" and go on with the marriage plans.

Sometime after their wedding, her new husband went back to see the doctor for a check-up. The doctor was baffled.

After further testing they determined that the *diagnosis had been wrong*. He didn't have ALS—it was Multiple Sclerosis, a much less fatal disease.

They put the florist business up for sale and made plans to move to the East Coast where Frank would be teaching at a university.

"Words cannot express how grateful we are to the Thompsons for sharing their story—it literally changed our life," she told Mom. "We will never forget you."

§

Troy has never stopped giving gifts to me, even after he has gone. Some I am still discovering in the lessons he taught and the legacy he left.

And on my birthday, one month after Troy died, I received a dozen roses…

…..this time a dozen white roses with one red.

Epilogue
STAIRWAYS AND TORCHES

"Whatever you can do, or dream you can, begin it.
Boldness has genius, power and magic in it."
~*Johan Wolfgang von Goethe*

Twelve years have passed since I wrote this book. That's a long time—a very long time. It deserves some explaining.

After Troy died, I knew I was going to need to take some time to heal, physically and emotionally. Now a widow with a young child, my demanding real estate career was no longer a good option. After working for another year or so, I left my career and spent the next year writing this book. Once it was finished, it was time to figure out what to do next.

As a result of much soul-searching and a series of divinely orchestrated events, the next journey of my life began with a new business. It was important to me to figure out a way to work from home to be with Victoria, and I wanted to do something to carry on our dream for the property, which was supposed to have been for Troy's landscaping business.

From this strong desire to start a home-based business that would enable me to use what I had learned about the importance of what we put in and on our bodies, use my business background, fuel my creative passions, and use my art education, *"Victoria's Lavender"* was born. That was over ten years ago, and I am so humbled to think about how this all came together into a successful business. I have been able to be involved in Victoria's life every step of the way (she's now in college pursuing her dream of working for the Yankees one day)! I have watched her grow into an amazing young woman with her father's legacy deeply imbedded in her. Each day I get to work in a business that is custom designed for my talents and passion, with a business model of employing other moms so that they can stay at home with their children, too. It has become a passion of mine to encourage other moms to do whatever it takes to be there for their kids. I love that I get to help provide an income as well as a creative outlet for moms.

My life continues to be "extraordinary," and the journey of launching and running this business as a single parent is full of stories of challenges, heartaches, joy and miracles — but those will have to wait for a future book!

§

The realization has slowly sunk in that this book has been waiting for *me* to be ready. Writing the book was therapeutic for sure, but it's difficult to share something so personal. Actually "releasing" the book is huge. On one hand, I needed to be able to "release" Troy, and share with the world the extraordinary story of this courageous man. These past two years have been a turning point where I finally came to the realization that Troy was in my life for a season, not a lifetime — and that there is still a lot of living to do.

On the other hand, I needed to know if it had God's blessing...if it was his desire to have the book published. If I could know that... well... that changes everything. If it was just my desire, then all kinds of doubts start to surface. What if it's not good enough? What if no one wants to read it except my closest friends?

If this book that had been on hold for twelve years was going to be released, I knew I would have to get a clear memo from above.

The "memo" came in a vision…

§

It was a long, expansive, white, sandy beach stretching in both directions as far as I could see. The ocean was calm, tiny waves curling onto the white sand at the water's edge. The sky was blue—not a cloud in sight. Behind me was a long, white, wooden staircase. I saw myself sitting alone on the beach, cross-legged in the sand. I was holding a book in my lap with both hands. Clutching it, really, not sure of what to do with it.

An angelic being appeared next to me. I never really saw his face, but he was dressed in white and gold. He asked me to give the book to him—to let it go, so it could be released. (Many times these past years I have pondered Habakkuk 2:2-3 where God tells the prophet, "Write down the revelation and make it plain on tablets so that a herald may run with it. For the revelation awaits an appointed time." I have asked God "Is it time? Is the runner going to come?")

I handed him the book and watched intently to see which way he would go—which of the three choices he would take. One choice was to go down the beach to the left, which stretched much farther than I could have walked. To the right, the beach also went as far as I could see and too far for me to go. Or would he go up the white wooden stairs? I didn't know what was at the top of those stairs, but was starting to become curious.

Instead, he didn't take any of those choices. He went up —and disappeared out of sight. And so did my book...

I sat there, wondering what was coming next. Was I supposed to do something?

After several minutes passed, I instinctively knew that I was supposed to go up those stairs. I started climbing, expecting to find a weathered beach house or maybe a road at the top.

Instead, when I reached the last step, I found myself at the top of a precipice. Looking over the edge, I was looking into a massive, bowl-shaped space. At first, I thought maybe it was a big sports stadium, but as the vision came into focus, I realized what I was seeing. It appeared to be the world with the top of it cut off so I could see into it. I could tell it was night because of the darkness punctuated by millions of lights, like the nightscape of a giant city.

As I stood there wondering what this all meant, the angel appeared beside me. He told me that those weren't lights of houses or buildings — they were lights like torches, lights from God's people that were "cities set on a hill" all over the world. The runner (angel) said that he was taking the book to light more torches.

And then the vision was over.

§

God showed me that not only was I ready, but the world was ready. It was significant that in the vision of the world it was night, darkness. He was showing me that the world needs the light that he has given each one of us, in unique ways. I am not to take the credit or glory for where the book goes, or what it does. Nor is the two-edged sword of pride to get in the way of it being released..."will it be good enough, what will people think, what if no one buys it?" That's partly why the angel took it from me.

So here it is, released out of my hands. Both excited and nervous at the same time, I look forward with great anticipation to hearing about the different torches that are lit throughout the world. May Troy's legacy of hope continue to be heard today around the world as it was in 1998. It's time...

§

Author's Note

The assisted suicide law, or "Death with Dignity Act," remains in effect in Oregon. In 2001, a federal law suit was filed against the state of Oregon in opposition to the Death with Dignity Act. After five years in the courts, it went all the way to the Supreme Court where it was upheld in 2006.

Since the law went into effect in 1997, the number of deaths in Oregon using the lethal prescriptions under the law has risen steadily. There were 77 know DWDA deaths in 2012 (source: Oregon Public Health Division Annual Report). Two more states — Washington and Montana — passed similar laws or rulings in 2009, and in May 2013, state lawmakers in Vermont approved a bill to legalize doctor-assisted suicide. Five additional states have similar bills being considered. There are only three countries in the world legalizing physician-assisted suicide.

As of this writing, there is still no treatment or cure for ALS.

APPENDIX
MANLY LIST

I. Seek first God with all your heart, mind, and soul.

II. Love your neighbor as you would yourself.

III. Prioritize each and every day: God first, family second, friends, work, and strangers (not forgetting the Church).

IV. Wake up believing that Jesus Christ is coming this very day to redeem His own!

V. Always let your "Yes" be yes and your "No" be no.

VI. Remember to love your wife "as Christ loved the church (gulp), He died for it!"

VII. Before adding one thing to your schedule, take away something else first! **

VIII. Every day, at least once a day, pray with your wife and read the Bible to her. You are the spiritual leader of your family. ***

IX. Our Lord God loves us enough to even rebuke us should we stray. Are not we to love our children just as much?

X. Remember, when praying, silence is not refusal. *

XI. Brother, in all these, walk in the Spirit and finish the race set before us.

XII. Mathematical equation to successful relationships... "Love = Time." *

XIII. This world is the closest thing to Hell a Christian will ever know...likewise this world is the closest thing to Heaven a sinner will ever know. ****

In Christ's love,
Troy N. Thompson
11/15/96

"Above all else, guard your heart,
For it is the wellspring of life."
Proverbs 4:23

* Pastor Ron
** Dr. James Dobson
*** Coach "PK" McCarthy
**** Dr. Roy Hicks, Sr.

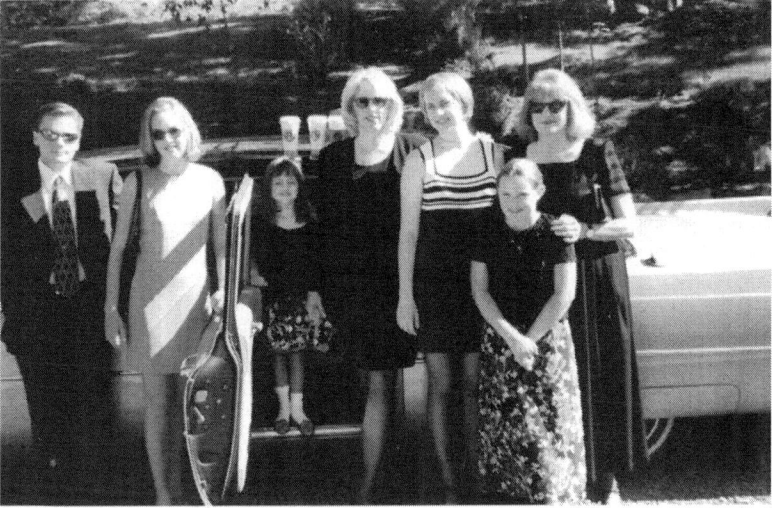

On our way to the funeral: Josh, Summer, Victoria, Marilyn, Holly, Marlene, and Michelle

Below ▼ Working four long days a week, Josh Henley has been Troy Thompson's caregiver for more than a year, part of a team of support that includes a hospice volunteer, night nurses, a social worker, family and friends. Henley's work and personal relationship with Thompson are credited with a dramatic improvement in his condition. "No one can do everything Josh can do," Marilyn Thompson said.

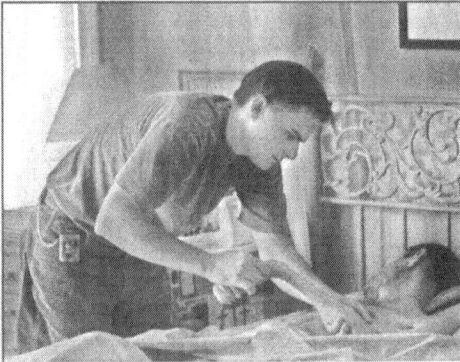

Josh

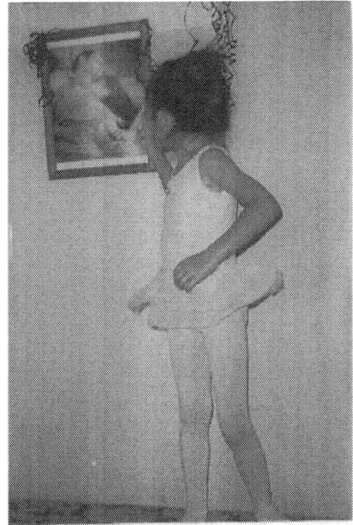

Victoria - 1998

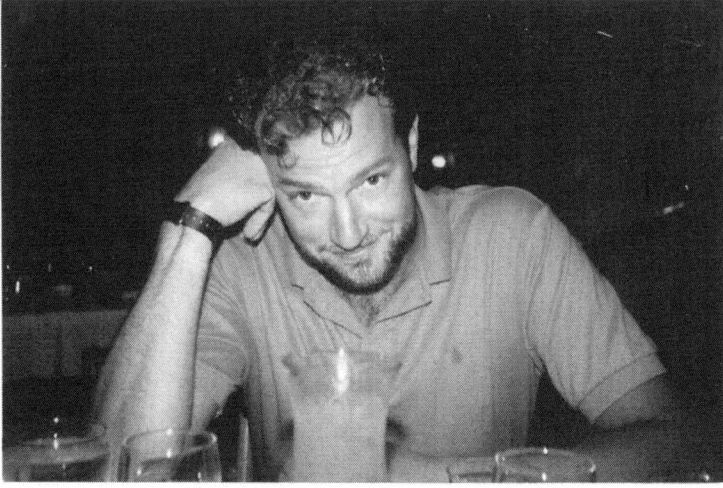

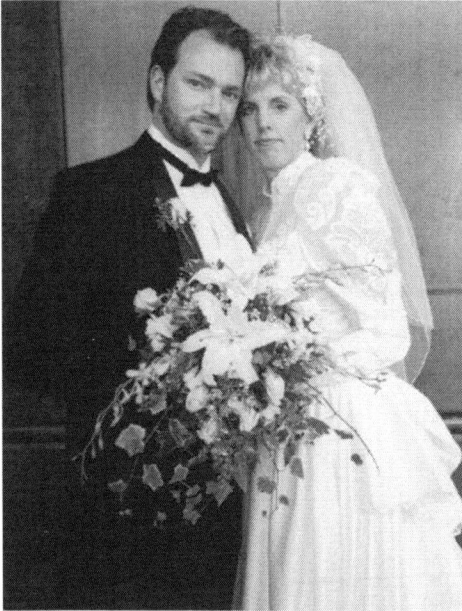

Married March 14, 1992

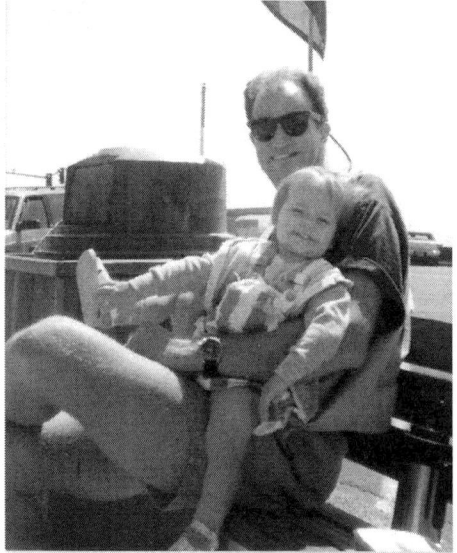

Just weeks before the diagnosis

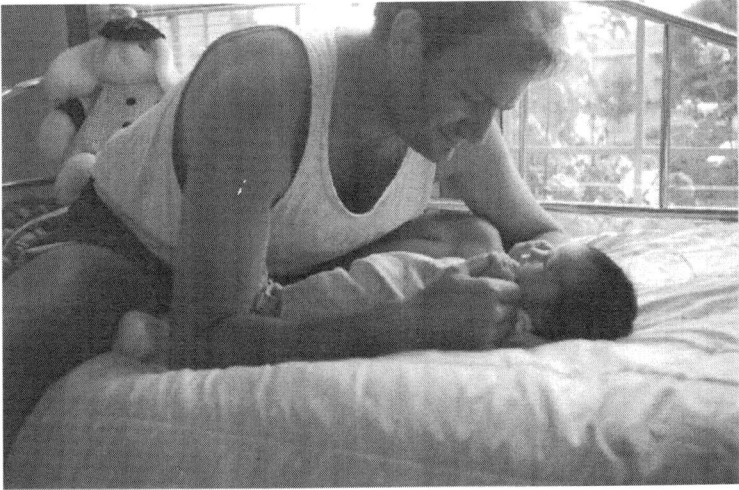

Victoria with her proud Papa at one month old

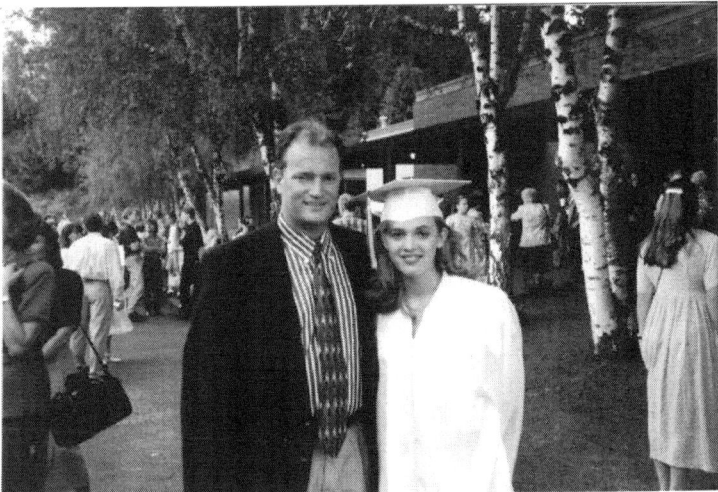

Summer's Graduation from Lake Oswego HS
June 1994, one month after the diagnosis

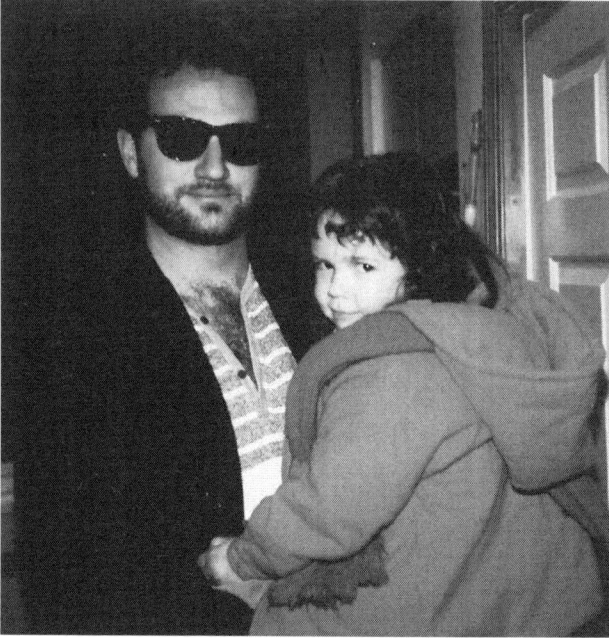
Troy and Michelle 1990

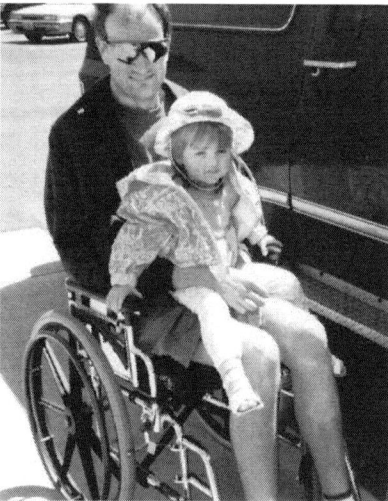
1994 with Victoria

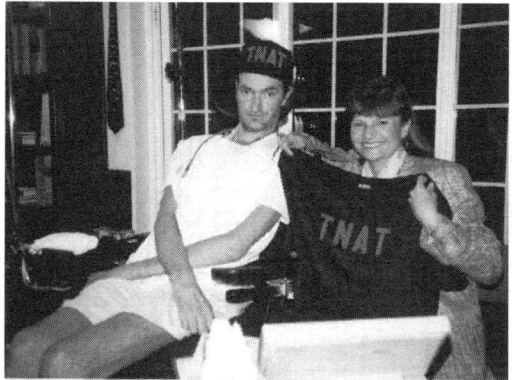
MaryBeth made Troy a shirt with his new middle initial: "A" for awesome

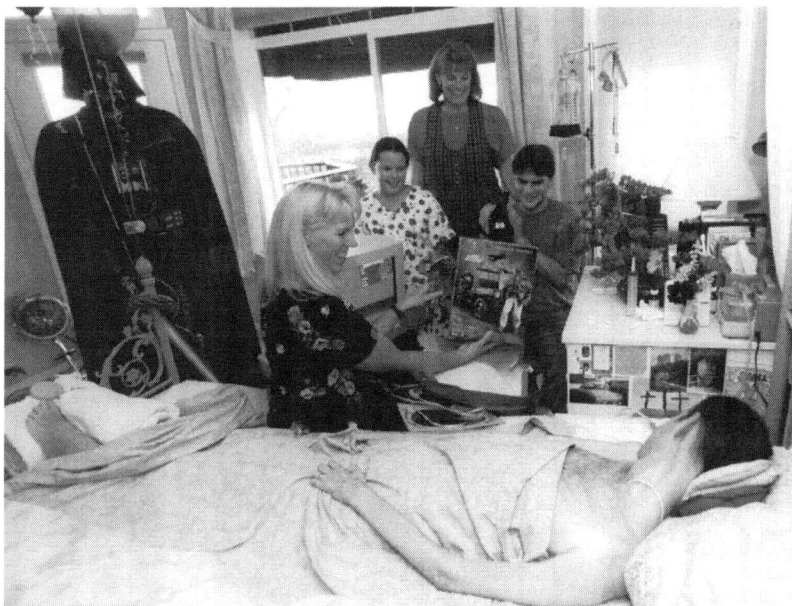

Another new GI Joe for his birthday!
(Marilyn, Michelle, Marlene and Josh)

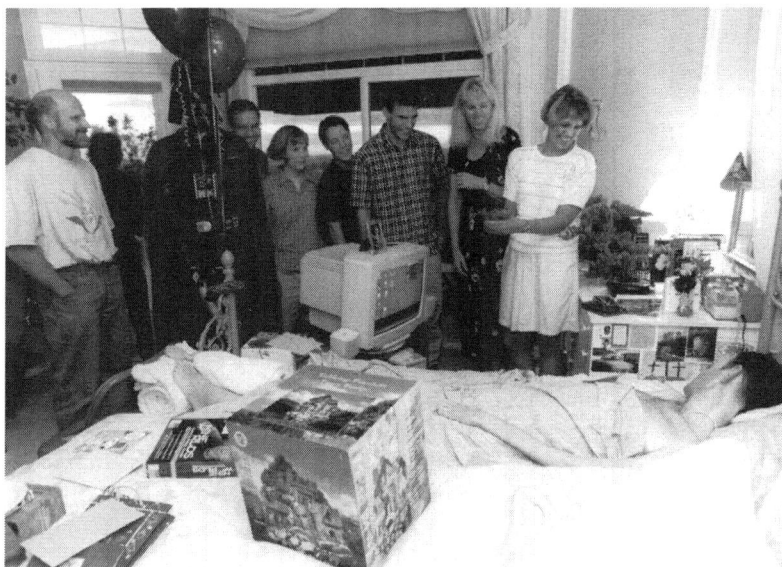

Troy's final Birthday Party
Left: Michael Sawyer plus the Williams' family

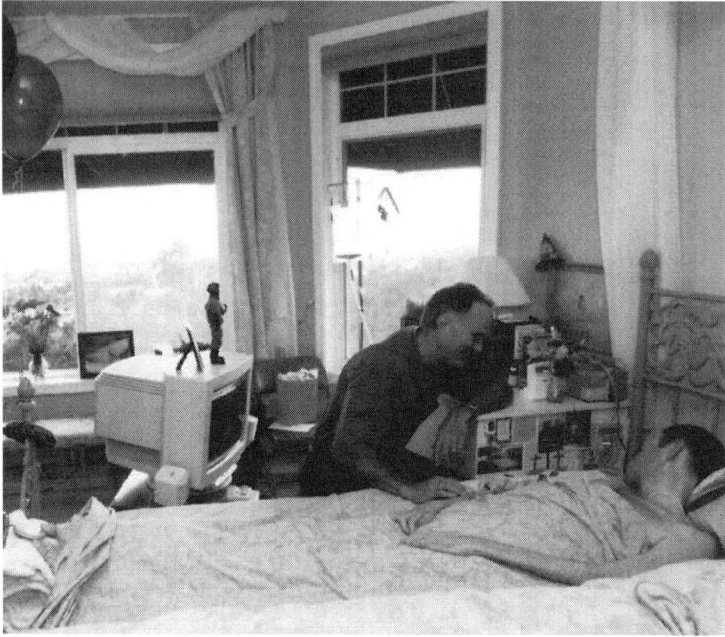

Bert Waugh, a regular visitor

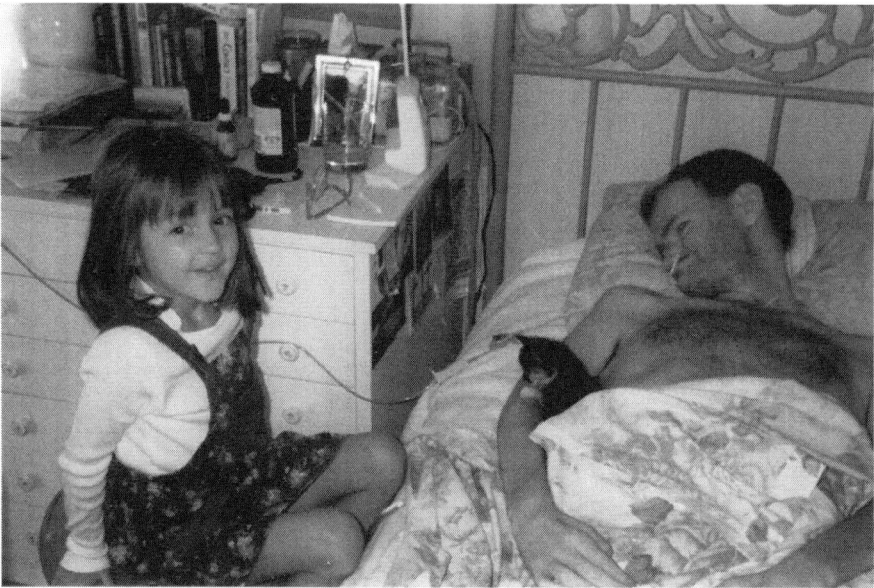

Troy sure enjoyed his daughters… and the kittens!

The girls loved to nap with their Dad

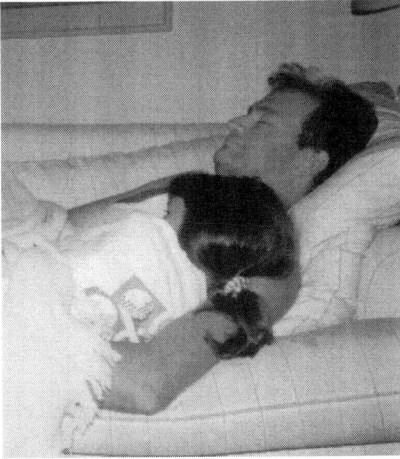

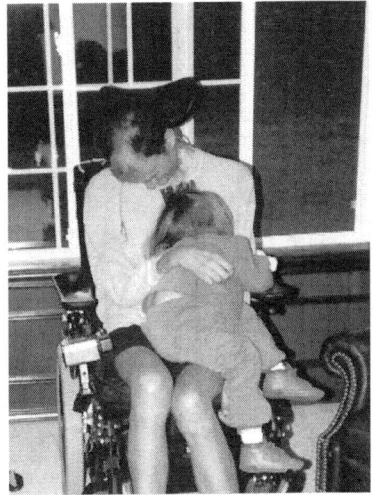

Michelle and Troy before the illness

3 year old Victoria

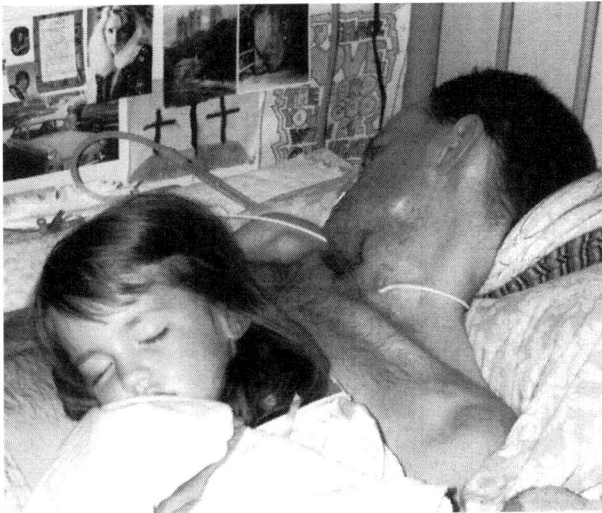

4 Year old Victoria

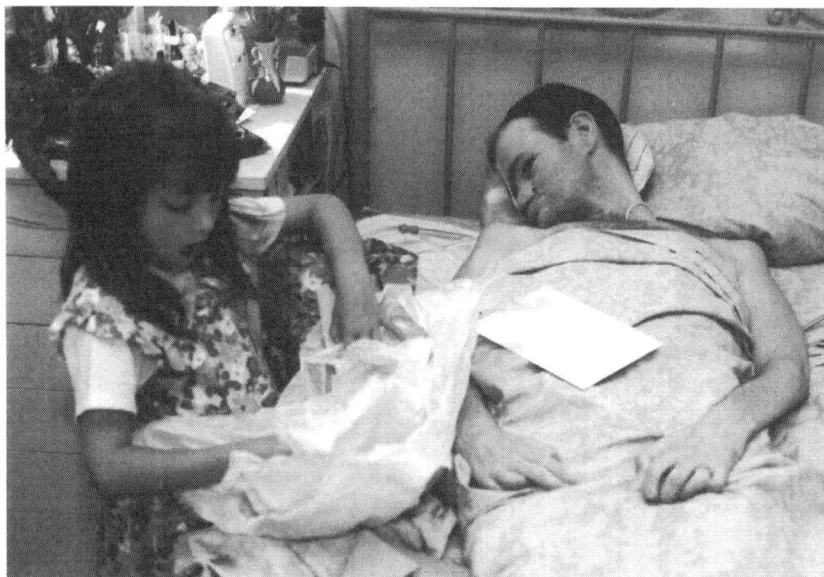

4 year old Victoria helping her Daddy open presents

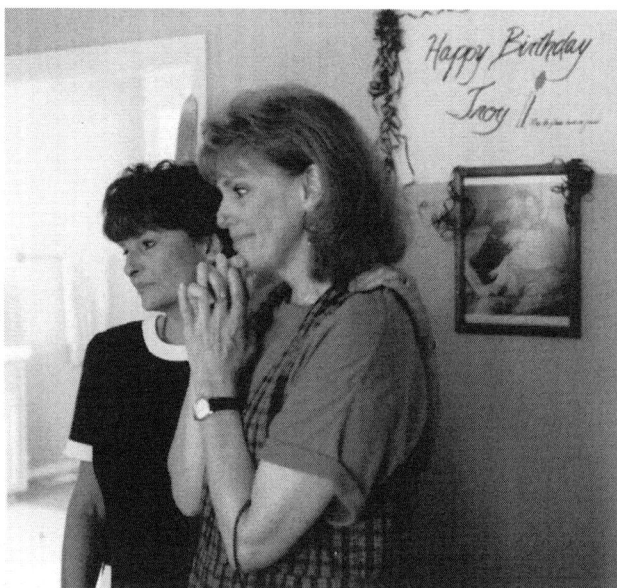

MaryBeth and Marlene watching Troy and Victoria

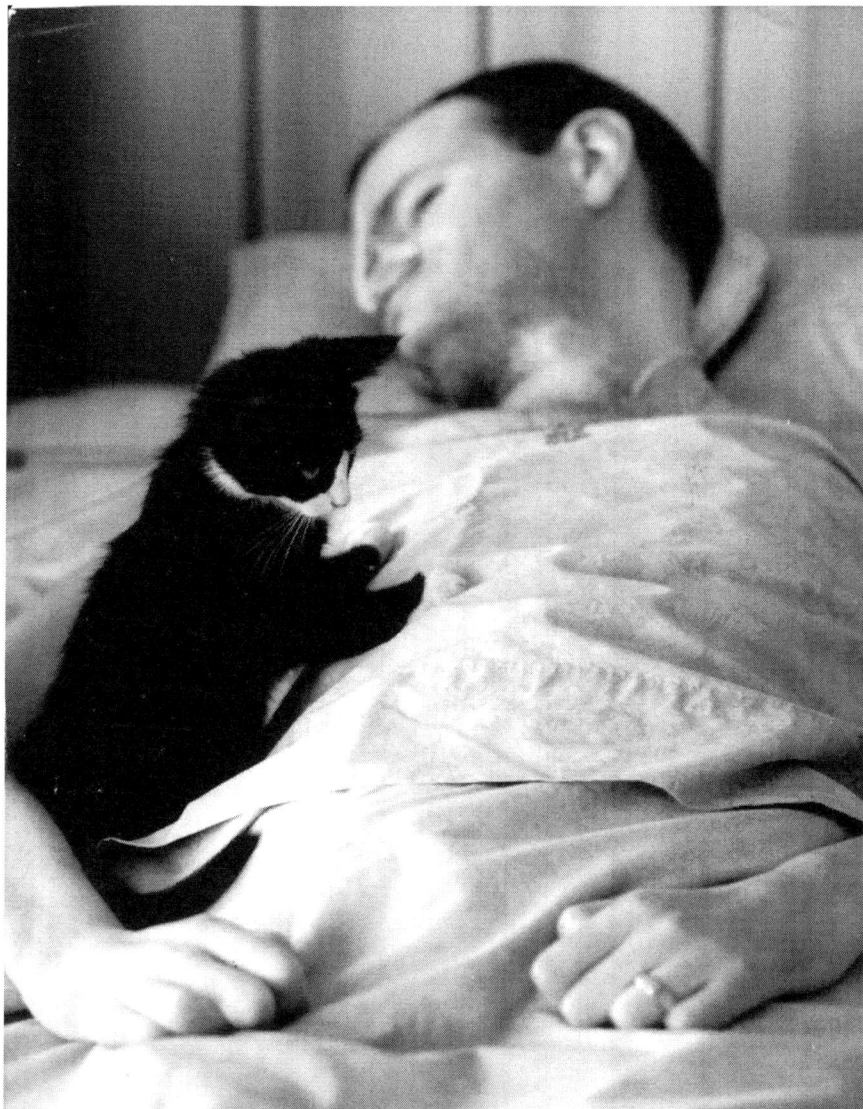

Oregonian Photo by Michael Lloyd
from top 10 stories for 1997

ACKNOWLEDGMENTS

Writing this book meant re-living the toughest years of my life—and some of the best, too. Walking back along that road and remembering all the hard times, the good times, the friends, the experiences…It was probably the best thing I could have done to allow myself to move forward and begin the healing process.

In turning this book into a reality, one person stands tall above the crowd…the late Dr. Ron Mehl. Without his continued encouragement throughout the writing process, I don't know that I would have forged ahead and believed that I could write something worthwhile.

A huge thank you to my editor, Elizabeth Jones, for providing the polish and to David Sanford for generously sharing his publishing knowledge along the way.

I am forever grateful to my daughters Summer, Holly, Michelle, and Victoria who, in each of their own ways, sacrificed part of their childhood. You girls were treasured in the individual ways you found to help out and to provide some "normalcy" to our family life. Also to Marlene, Troy's Mom, who remained steadfast and strong, faithfully caring for Victoria on weekends and providing a vital extra set of hands, always putting others needs ahead of her own.

There were so many, many people that came alongside us during those four years to help in a variety of ways that our family will be forever grateful for. Pastor Keith Reetz from Beaverton Foursquare was a regular visitor and incredible prayer support. He was a calm in the storm so many times. Lucy and Mike Sawyer sacrificially poured out their time and friendship to be with us every step of the way. Bert Waugh was one of our pillars of strength and there were times I'm not sure how we would have made it through without Bert being there to support us. Josh Henley, Troy's full time caregiver, was the glue that held us together, on the front lines day after day, loyal and faithful, invaluable beyond description.

A special thanks to Mark O'Keefe and the staff at the Oregonian; so many great doctors like Dr. Wendy Johnston and the late Dr. Miles Edwards; the ALS center at OHSU; my "Breakfast Club" friends Geri Warmanen, Kathy Goeddel, and MaryBeth Baker, also ALS widows whose husbands had all passed on before Troy; and our wonderful neighbors here in Newberg. Thank you to Troy's many caregivers including Marvina Coleman, Diane Cooper, Janice Van Tassel Taisey, and the hospice staff and volunteers—you all gave so much selfless and loving care.

Thank you to the people we worked with at Prudential Northwest Properties and Marion County. Your kindness and flexibility helped us navigate our challenges to continue working.

Thank you to my prayer group that has stayed steadfast and always there for me and my family these past fifteen years—Gayleen Weiler, Gary Gorsuch, Michael Beirwagen, and Bert Waugh.

Thank you to so many more friends and family members, to churches and individuals, some of whom I've never met, that prayed for us, wrote letters, did yard work, made financial contributions, cooked meals, and a host of other contributions.

And finally, to the prayer warriors from Co-Labor Ministry along with the Bethel team of students from Redding as well as Elrike Shaw that helped me to realize that the time had come to launch this book.

Thank you all…from the bottom of my heart.

ABOUT THE AUTHOR

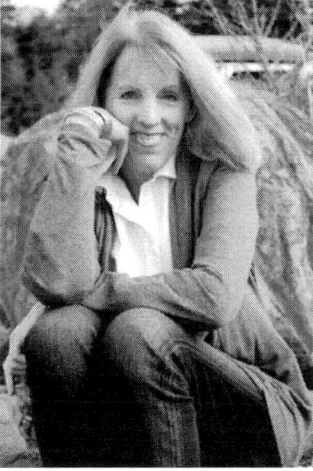

Marilyn Thompson was born in Portland, Oregon, and currently resides in the hills of Newberg in Oregon's wine country. She is the creator and owner of Victoria's Lavender, LLC, named after their youngest daughter. The lavender is grown on the property she and Troy purchased together, one month before his diagnosis. Marilyn is the proud mother of four daughters—Summer, Holly, Victoria, and step-daughter Michelle plus son-in-laws Jay and Sean, and grandsons Jackson and Joseph.

If after reading this book you are impacted by the story and would like to share your comments, please email them to comments@marilynthompson-author.com or post them on the author's blog at marilynthompson-author.com.

Marilyn can be found on her websites at:
www.marilynthompson-author.com
www.victoriaslavender.com

She can also be found on her Facebook pages at:
facebook.com/MarilynThompson-Author and
Facebook.com/VictoriasLavender.
The twitter accounts are @victoriaslavndr and
@mthompsonauthor